Walking Ella

Robert Drewe

To Laura,

who walks her least
and loves her most

Walking Ella

Ruminations of a
reluctant dog-walker

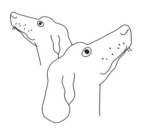

Robert Drewe

VIKING
an imprint of
PENGUIN BOOKS

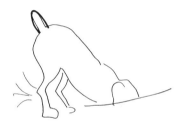

It's a humid, dusty Sunday in Centennial Park and I'm
being poked in the chest by a man who is shouting at me,
so furious that tears are spurting from his eyes like bullets.

'Your evil dog is giving my wife post-natal depression!'
he yells.

The man is Indian, I think, and so agitated that he is
producing projectile tears. His lips are trembling. My small

son grips my hand in fright as the man keeps prodding me. As I try to dodge his poking finger, picnickers watch us with interest. Everyone's attention has been caught by the man's shouts, by women's wailing and arm-waving and the flurry of saris.

If only I could turn the clock back ten minutes. Way back then, dog, boy and father were lolling in the farthest, shadiest, dog-permitted reaches of the park. And then on the faintest of summer breezes, across the competing smells of the bumper-to-bumper traffic on the park's ring road and the pungent horse-riding track and five or six hundred metres of swampy lake and recently mown grass, to her alone of all the dogs and people here, wafted the aroma of distant curry.

And she was off.

Now Ella's mouth is greasy with dhal and poppadom crumbs. She darts around us, swerving from my lunging hands. Her body surges and twists with the thrill of the hubbub. She's charged by the family's hysteria, transformed into something white-eyed and crazy and rippling like a nervy racehorse. It's as if all her springy litheness has been bred into her just for this perfect moment of chaos.

No one comprehends my apologetic dog-logic. *I'm very sorry. Please relax. Ignore her. Believe me, your screaming and jumping is just exciting her. She doesn't bite. She's just playful.*

I feel total, one hundred per cent sympathy. The Indian woman has a young baby. My dog is wrecking a peaceful family gathering.

Let's be honest, there's also a small but growing annoyance at the finger jabs and wild theatrics. But I feel so guilty I can't yell at them, *Get a grip!* (Would I be so passive if these were *wurst*-munching Germans, say, picnicking in *lederhosen*, prodding me?)

Anyway, no one's listening to me. Not the Indians, certainly not Ella. It's like shouting in a dream. I'm standing there sweating and bewildered, in a familiar agitated trance. The situation is now far beyond dog and people and a disrupted picnic and differing East/West attitudes to pets. It's deep, dark, collective-unconscious stuff now, genetics and myth and the shadow of the hawk. Or wolf.

Of course Ella's to blame again, once more an agent of turbulence and disarray.

She might look like a dog – a handsome, liver-coloured, spayed, German shorthaired pointer bitch – but she's actually a sort of anti-dog. She doesn't fetch or come, or even favour a particular person. While she probably prefers our family to strangers, she'll betray us for anyone with a bag of chips or a ham sandwich.

Granted, an optimistic beckoning whistle does sometimes stop her in her tracks – then just as we're heaping astonished congratulations on her she'll toss her head and gallop the other way. I fear she's unlikely to change. She's six years old – middle-aged, for God's sake.

Perhaps, as the Indian man insists, she is 'evil'. Dogs are a symbol of evil in some mythologies. But her drives are more simple, and complex, than that. She's ruled by her nose, by her breed's bloodhound genes. To smell is potentially to eat, and she lives to eat. She'll eat anything that can't be strictly classified as mineral. And at the moment her whole reason for existence hinges on those poppadoms and curries.

Despite my entreaties, the Indian family won't calm down. They won't stop shouting and jumping about. The woman, who has now begun to howl, holds her baby horizontally above her head, as if from a tiger or a wolf. The baby is beginning to scream, and an older, plumper, moaning woman, presumably the grandmother, is trying to take it from its mother.

Grandmother has climbed onto a drinks cooler. She's wobbling on the cooler's lid and yelling for the mother to pass the baby over her head to her for safety in case Ella devours them both. But the mother refuses to give it up, so they wrestle over it for a while, wailing and keening, while Ella barks and leaps joyfully at them.

I'm aware of the muttering and movement of the other picnickers. Egged on by their wives, men in their weekend shorts and baseball caps get up from their picnics, some holding cricket bats and sticks, and start towards us. They're saying, 'What's going on here?'

Denied the baby, the grandmother has come to the decision to bravely sacrifice herself. She clambers down from the drinks cooler, rushes at the dog in a flurry of silks, and starts pelting her with cutlery and food containers. This really sets Ella barking with excitement. She can't believe the high standard of entertainment, especially with spicy food thrown in.

Meanwhile, the younger woman is standing on her toes and holding the baby so high above her head that her sari exposes more than her midriff. The shouts of her husband become shriller and the baby cries louder.

And, fighting against the sensation that I'm actually in a dream, I finally break the stalemate. Abruptly, I break and run.

I'm turning my back on these people who hate me and my dog, on the whole picnic-ground fracas. I'm also performing the only known successful method of getting Ella to come.

I grab up my son, run across the park to my car, jump in and speed away. I brake sharply after about fifty metres, sound the horn, then speed off once more, again beeping the horn. I stop and start a few more times. By now the whole picnic ground is standing and pointing at our jerky, honking progress.

And then I slow down as Ella, disconcerted that her fed-up 'master' has finally decided to leave her for ever, makes the decision to forgo the poppadoms. She knifes across the park like a greyhound, through the crowds of cursing picnickers, and jumps into the moving getaway car.

Once again I despair of Ella. All her life, she and her daily walk have been the fulcrum of my working day.

Her 'walk' is a compulsory and often unwelcome interruption. I begrudge her my time and, even more, my loss of choice. She eats a lot and needs vigorous exercise. So do I. My preference is for swimming. I'd rather be swimming at Bondi than trudging around the park. But this ninety minutes is all I can spare each day, and dogs are forbidden on Sydney's beaches. So my only time off is not my own.

This would be acceptable, however, if she behaved. If she actually 'walked'. If, having gambolled and galloped and frolicked as much as she liked, she then returned. If she

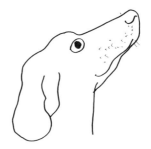

It feels very strange
and ironic
trying to capture her
frequent look of nobility.

This angle is actually
the one she uses for
human-bottom sniffing

didn't run for her life, head for the hills, once it was time to leave. If she didn't create embarrassing, disgusting havoc. If she – this is pathetic now – listened to me.

Anyway, the Indian picnic disaster makes me take stock. As my wife points out, blithely farewelling the pair of us next morning, 'We're stuck with her.' That's not good enough for me: to hand over my life, every vestige of control, to a dog. A dog, I might add, presently lounging on the sofa like some spoiled empress, farting away yesterday's curry lunch, and earlier brunch of possum cadaver, and eyeing me with a jaundiced glance somewhere between dyspepsia and ennui.

So, like a prisoner with a long sentence in front of him, I decide I can do my time hard or easy. It occurs to me that it might be cathartic to write a dog-walker's journal: the true, unsentimental ruminations of a dog-walker with things on his mind more important than dogs. A dog-walker who, frankly, prefers humans. A dog-walker who decides to make the most of this begrudged walk to mull over writing ideas and dilemmas. A prickly, grumpy, even sometimes hungover dog-walker.

I'll consider her in the context of dogs in general, in the reality of her, and my, daily surroundings – Centennial Park – and my domestic and working life.

It's only just registering how important the park has been to me for a long while. It's where my wife and I have wooed and canoodled and strolled and argued and negotiated and exercised and relaxed. Tears and sweat have been shed here, and – on the bike and horse tracks – a little blood. It's where I walk with my daughters to discuss Life. We've all eaten many picnic sandwiches here, kicked many footballs, fed many ducks. We've held birthday parties here, watched hockey games and two codes of football and many primary-school sports days. (Who could forget the legendary 1984 girls' 12-years-and-under 800 metres event where a sort of contagious frenzy, similar to the girls' hysteria in *The Crucible*, mysteriously swept over the competitors, leaving them wheezing and writhing on the ground? Except for a little eight-year-old entrant, running a lap behind and thus immune from the mass panic attack, who trotted around the heaving bodies and came home as winner.)

By collating Ella's habits and revealing her disgusting secrets, perhaps I can even exact a sort of revenge. ('This is where you fit in, Ella!') Instead of the usual sentimental tripe about a man and his loyal canine pal, these would be the realistic ramblings of someone daily driven to distraction by his dog.

You see, Ella is not a dog of Christmas calendars or chocolate-tin lids or hunting prints. She isn't this man's best friend, nor has she lowered his blood pressure, as dogs are famously supposed to do for their owners. (I wouldn't dare take my blood pressure after our walks – even on those times when we manage to arrive home together.)

Best of all, she'll be working for her living. Yes, there is a strange satisfaction in the idea of keeping a dossier on Ella.

My children begged for a dog and, of all the pups in the litter, for her. They were actively encouraged by my English-born wife, whose Cotswold childhood of horses and green Hunter Wellingtons had imbued in her a need for muddy dogs underfoot and with first claim to the comfiest chairs. (Whereas my Australian childhood dogs were not allowed indoors and thought themselves lucky to sleep in the laundry.)

A familiar story: I was the only one of the family who didn't want another dog and now the dog and I spend our days together.

I walk her and feed her. And as I scrub the various manures and the stink of decayed possum corpse from her fur, as (my own gorge rising) I scoop out those indescribably obscene disgorgements and excretions from the back seat of my car, I wonder yet again where are those pleading dog-lovers now?

P.1

ABC RADIO

3LO 774

Australian
Broadcasting
Corporation

ABC Southbank Centre
Southbank Boulevard
Southbank
Victoria 3006

GPO Box 9994
Melbourne 3001

Tel (03) 9624 1600
Fax (03) 9626 1774

FAX COVER SHEET

TO:

Attention:	MARIA FOR R. DREWE
Organisation:	"PAN MACMILLAN"
Fax number:	(02) 9261 5047
Date / time:	THURSDAY

CONTACT DETAILS:

From:	JULIANNE PAGE
	ABC Radio, 3LO.
Fax:	(03) 9626 1774
Phone:	(03) 9626 1759

Number of pages including cover sheet: 1.

Additional message:

Dear Maria —

This fax is to confirm interview between ABC Sunday Arts presenter Sian Prior and author Robert Drewe on Sunday March 22nd at 12.10 pm. A Sydney "Tardis Booth" has been booked for Robert at ABC Ultimo from 12 noon. The interview will go (approx) 10 minutes and we would appreciate him being at Ultimo by 12 noon. Sian has read "The Drowner" and is looking forward to talking to Robert about this. Any queries? Please call me on (03) 9626 1759

Julianne Page

//

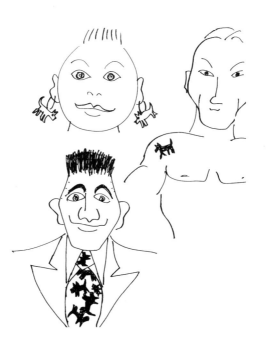

It's not as if I'm not used to dogs. My family has owned five dogs before Ella. Four of them were sensible animals. They weren't canine paragons, but they were sound in head and body and reasonably well-behaved.

They knew their place (a bed in the laundry), and made no enemies. No man ever accused Shandy or Monty or Charlie of giving his wife post-natal depression.

But the first of these five dogs was a sad case. He was a border-collie/collie cross I was given when I was ten. I'd been pestering my mother for a dog for four or five years. I'd seen this mournful pup in the pet-shop window. Finally she gave in, and eventually talked my father around.

I named the pup Shep, after the fictional loyal collie. But this trustworthy sheepdog's name gave him no confidence. He was highly-strung and easily offended, with his unfortunate pet-shop background and hurt eyes.

Despite his soft coat and snooty nose, Shep lacked both a collie's aloof briskness and a border-collie's working-class geniality. He slunk apologetically around the yard, too readily convinced he was the lowest member of the pack. He dug apathetic shallow holes in the dirt and lay in them. The cat bossed him around. His behaviour was the canine equivalent of tugging his forelock and calling you guv'nor. He was insincerely subservient. If he could have talked he would have made bitter jokes about his pet-shop origins.

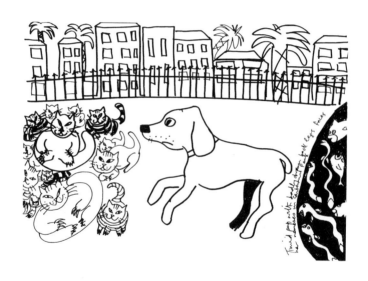

14

Romantically, I tried to imagine him differently. I deeply denied my disappointment with him. He was my dog and I loved him. Did part of me think this was compulsory? I certainly saw us as an adventurous boy and his heroic dog in a movie. I wanted him to snap out of it and save people from floods and fires and shipwrecks and be on the newsreels.

———————————

One day when Shep was twelve months old, and my back was turned, he was 'sent to the country'. That afternoon they told me his hurt eyes had been weeping pus. He was cringing around the yard even more listlessly than usual, they alleged, and had nipped my sister, although there was no mark on her that convinced as evidence. The man in the pet shop had lied about his distemper innoculation.

When I got home from school it was too late. Shep was already in the country. Although no one would come clean (nor, for some reason, could I closely question them), I knew from the solemn manner of their announcement, and the way they kept looking at me, what the euphemism meant. The country was death.

Maybe a canine-inclined shrink would say my response to Ella stems from my never recovering from Shep's being sent to the country.

Shep's brief existence broke the parental ice about dogs. When the next one made its appearance my brother claimed him, and I didn't object. I didn't want to love another dog and lose him to the country.

This was Shandy, a sort of gingery, elongated variation on a Jack Russell. Shandy's name, my father's idea, was regarded in the family as clever, suiting both his variegated beer-and-lemonade colouring as well as his being a mixture.

He was a bouncy, unassuming little fellow. He'd come running with me. I was training for athletics and before breakfast I'd run along Perth's Swan River shore, past the Sunset old men's home and through the bamboo thickets and along the beachfront to the Nedlands jetty and back. Shandy would generally find a dead blowfish on the beach, discarded from a prawner's net, and so stiff it crackled in his teeth, and carry it home to savour at his leisure.

This made him unpopular with my mother, who was forever finding these stinking bits of blowfish parchment around the house. But then my mother died suddenly one afternoon while still young, and in the chaos that followed we sort of forgot about Shandy.

I remember that in my father's anguished attempts to recover domestic equilibrium (the hiring and firing of housekeepers, the late-night consumption of Dewar's) that Shandy was given to friends. And for the first time in thirty years, it occurs to me, with a cold rush, while writing these notes that 'given to friends' (which friends? where?) was another euphemism of my father's.

———————————

Monty made an appearance about a year later, my sister's dog this time. Monty was mostly Welsh corgi.

The family says that Monty was around for about ten years. That I have no recollection whatsoever of his personality says more of my dislocation from the family at this time than of Monty's lack of character.

———————————

Ella was named by my second daughter after a school friend who had gone to live in America. My daughter missed her friend Ella and liked her name.

A year later a female acquaintance was at our place for lunch. Noting Ella's name and rich brown colouring ('liver-coloured', in the breeding books), the woman said suddenly, 'Isn't that racist?'

'What?' I said.

'Ella Fitzgerald,' she said smugly.

As it happened, our new next-door neighbour shortly after married an African-American woman. We invited them over for coffee. Ella was very much underfoot, between people's legs as usual, sniffing bottoms. All the family was exasperatedly calling out her name.

I suddenly felt stupidly embarrassed. Did the woman stiffen when she heard Ella's name or did I imagine it?

She's the first pure-bred dog we've owned, and the hungriest. If they're such European aristocrats, wouldn't you think they'd have some polite restraint bred into them? She has no cut-off mechanism with food. If tasty food kept coming she would eat until she exploded.

You can tell when she has been stealing food because it forms an immediate incriminating roll of fat around her neck and shoulders. If the breeze is right she can smell food more than a kilometre away. I use the word 'food' loosely. I mean everything from a drunk's vomit outside the Windsor Castle to stolen Thai leftovers or a road-killed cat.

After a particularly hot curry her nose stays dry and hot for a day and she looks at you as if you've hurt her feelings. She seems to be requiring an apology. Nonetheless she can't resist the green Thai curry served at the Bellevue Hotel, whose bins she raids whenever she escapes from the back yard. Further afield, the Sri Lankan curry at the London Tavern

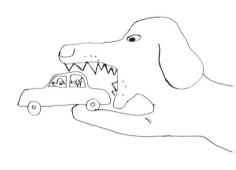

and the pita breads and baba ganoush which the Lebanese
birdlover leaves in Queens Park are also perfectly acceptable.

Once, feeling especially attentive, I bought her an expensive
delicacy called Rover's Treat from the Woollahra butcher.
Choice lean beef. An hour later she vomited the Rover's
Treat up on the back seat of the car. She preferred a plastic
bag of decaying meat she found in one of the park's ponds an
hour later. Of course that stayed down. Indeed, it passed all
the way through, plastic shopping bag and all, the familiar
trademark houndstooth check of David Jones peeping out
the other end remarkably quickly.

During all this frustration I was doing more than just
planning writerly revenge on Ella. We were taking
conscientious dog owners' direct action, booking her in for
professional obedience training (it seemed appropriate when
we chanced upon a German trainer) and reading all the
current wisdom on both training and canine behaviour.

The book that made the biggest impression on me was
Leader of the Pack, subtitled *How to Take Control of Your
Relationship with Your Dog*, by the American dog lovers and
'experienced animal behaviourists' Nancy Baer and Steve
Duno. It was the stated intention of Nancy and Steve to
teach me 'to create an atmosphere that mirrored the
dynamics of a wolf pack'.

My home would become the wilderness. Number 118 would be a perfect tundra. More than that. Nancy and Steve promised to turn me into the Alpha Wolf of the household pack.

But before they did so they had a check-list of questions to shame me into realising how far down the wolf-pack order I was cringing at the moment.

Did I let my dog go through doors ahead of me? *Yes.* Did I serve her dinner before I ate my own? *Yes.* Did she greet visitors before I did? *Yes.* Did she successfully bump my hand to get petted? *Yes.* Did she pull ahead of me on the lead? *Of course.* Did I let her win tugs-of-war? *Yes.* Did I let her choose the time and place for relieving herself? *I suppose so.* Did I have to repeat commands to get her to listen? *Are you kidding?* Did she sleep on our bed? *Hardly.* Did she protest if I tried to cut her nails? *What?*

Well, I scored two out of ten. I'd never permitted her on our bed and, frankly, trimming her nails hadn't occurred to me. Obviously I was only a Gamma Wolf at best.

———————

I discovered that the first German shorthaired pointer was registered in German Kennel Club stud books in 1872. The breed had existed for some years before, as the product of various crosses between the old Spanish pointer and the

German bloodhound, with infusions from time to time of English and black pointers.

According to *The German Shorthaired Pointer*, edited by Diane McCarty, the exact number of crosses and recrosses can't be determined, 'for all of this has become hidden in the shroud of obscurity'.

The breed wasn't an overnight success. German huntsmen were dissatisfied with the scenting ability of the first German pointers and turned to hound crosses to improve the 'nose'. Early photographs show the shorthair as still having a very jowly hound appearance. Later, greater speed, 'nose' and more physical attractiveness were demanded (less floppy dewlaps), and breeders turned to good English pointers.

By the turn of the century, German breeders had almost reached their goal. 'They had formulated standards of physical perfection,' says McCarty. 'The Teutonic mind has never been easily satisfied, and as their dog's efficiency improved, their standards for perfection were lifted accordingly. With efficiency has come greater physical beauty based on sounder structure.'

In the Germans' eyes, however, one doggy bit still stuck out and marred this perfection. So they lopped it off. Unlike English pointers' tails, the shorthair's tail is docked to one-third its natural length. As McCarty diplomatically, and somewhat ludicrously, points out: 'This creates a trim appearance, prevents injury, from being caught going in or out of doors of cars and homes, and prevents the bloody sores that usually occur when a dog of active tail motion slashes it against trees and bushes during a day's hunt.'

Shorthair colouration is varied and ranges from solid liver to liver-and-roan, to liver-and-white. 'Any combination of liver and white is acceptable,' says McCarty, going on to say that 'the dog's short, tight coat is a virtue appreciated by the lady of the household, for it does not shed readily.'

As for temperament, the breed was all smooth sailing. 'The breed's cornerstone has been set on solid ground, and the shorthair is here to stay.' This paragon of virtue was powerful yet agile, of medium height and weight, large enough for any work required, and yet not so big as to be cumbersome in modern homes or cars.

'The shorthair's tractability has gained him many supporters from the ranks of men who have wearied of attempts to train or handle some of our stronger-headed gun dog breeds.'

All in all, 'the German shorthaired pointer's physical characteristics impress one as being those of an honest and energetic workman.'

Could we possibly have been thinking of the same breed? This thought, among others, flashed through my mind as

I accelerated away from the Dog and Master Obedience School, leaving behind the emotionally exhausted (German) dog trainer and his darkly furious female assistant. Through the rear-vision mirror I could see the woman still shaking her fist at us until our car rounded a bend in the road and she disappeared.

Three weeks as a boarder at the school run by the German trainer and his angry offsider and Ella could now, as the trainer demonstrated, Sit, Lie Down, Stay and Heel. For five seconds. If she was on a lead. Or perhaps within a metre of you. Otherwise forget it. He hadn't managed to convince her to Come or Fetch. Coming and Fetching, it's unnecessary to point out, are supposedly the chief skills of German shorthaired pointers. They're world-beaters at Coming and Fetching. (According to *Your Ideal Dog*, they score top points for 'trainability'.)

'Very difficult dog,' he'd whispered, running trembling fingers through his crewcut.

She'd also learned a dislike of any men outside the family and a fear of any object, from an umbrella to a cricket bat, that could be construed as a stick.

But she was certainly pleased to see us.

It's going too far to suggest that Ella was responsible for the German dog trainer appearing to be having a nervous breakdown and the dark woman being so full of rage that she was nudging insanity.

It was clear that these doggy people, living in the sparsely-populated outer-suburban wasteland of old car bodies, agistment paddocks, plant nurseries and boarding kennels, the thrum of the high-voltage power pylons and the interstate expressway always in their ears, were going mad. It was just unfortunate – let's be fair – that Ella's and their lives had crossed during this process.

When we'd dropped her off at the Dog and Master School three weeks before, they'd been friendly and pleasantly professional. Crisply dressed in efficient safari-style khaki. As Teutonically confident as the breeders of Ella's own ancestors. As they showed us around, several other canine clients had barked confidently but politely from their pens.

When we picked her up the trainers were wild-eyed and disshevelled. Their lives seemed to have disintegrated. And Ella appeared to be the only dog on the premises. What was the reason for the change? What had gone so wrong in three weeks? Trying to find the Dog and Master School again, we'd got lost out there beyond the road-guide, among those tussocky paddocks, sway-backed old horses and signs saying 'Chook Poo $2'. We'd arrived an hour later than anticipated.

GERMAN SHORTHAIRED POINTER

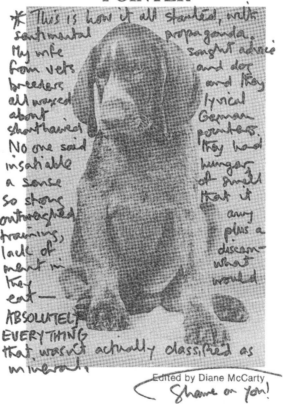

* This is how it all started, with sentimental propaganda. My wife sought advice from vets and dog breeders and they all waxed lyrical about German shorthaired pointers. No one said they had insatiable hunger, a sense of small so strong that it outweighed any training, plus a lack of discern-ment in what they would eat — ABSOLUTELY EVERYTHING that wasn't actually classified as mineral,

Edited by Diane McCarty

Shame on you!

There was another reason for our lateness. I was driving very cautiously. I'd just picked up my wife and new baby from the hospital. We'd sensibly timed Ella's three-week absence for the last days of pregnancy and the time of the baby's arrival. The idea was that the baby and the newly tranquil Ella would be coming home together.

As we blithely pulled up, the woman strode up to our car and abused us. She was a storm cloud of darkness and hatred. She peered through the car window at the tiny bundle and yelled at my wife, 'I'm sorry for him having been born to a bitch like you.' Even for someone whose skills were tightly concentrated in the area of canine rather than human relations this seemed extravagant abuse to heap on a customer – and one who hadn't paid yet.

'Don't think you're getting your dog back!' she screamed.

The man limply waved her away and ushered us into his office. 'Sorry,' he sighed but elaborated no further. 'Of course you will have your dog back.' He looked at me. 'You will find of course that Ella goes to you more than to your wife. She has more respect for your maleness. It's your hormone smell.'

I think this was meant as a compliment. (The old Alpha Wolf strikes again!) Whatever, his manner was that of someone under intense pressure. He was having as much difficulty forming sentences as we, still stunned and seething from the woman's tirade, were having in concentrating on them.

As he muttered briefly about Ella's 'training', he was also distractedly urging us to buy a lifetime's supply of dry dog pellets at cost price. He kept casting anxious glances through the office window as if at any minute he expected the woman to burst in waving an axe. His manner, if not his flattery about my smell, beseeched me not to cancel my cheque the moment we were off the premises.

The mystery of his assistant's flaming anger towards my wife (presumably my hormones saved me from a similar attack), and their erratically changed behaviour, niggled at me for a week or so. I even considered writing a short story about them. Then the image of the angry dog-woman running down the road after our car gradually faded and, as so often happens, the impetus for the story fell away.

———————————

I'm wondering vaguely whether I've ever used dogs in a story or novel.

At first I don't think so. Then I remember the Great Danes in the first novel, *The Savage Crows*, Dan Kelly's dog in *Our Sunshine*, the Rottweilers in the short story, 'Machete'. The Great Danes were imaginary but those Rottweilers were real. So, incidentally, was the mysterious machete I found in my front yard one morning.

I also used a real cat once, in *The Savage Crows* in a walk-on part. Jimpy. Jimpy followed me home from Bentleigh East primary school in Melbourne when I was five. Jimpy transferred with us to Western Australia a year later, lived to fourteen, and in his loyalty and obedience was actually a much better 'dog' than Ella.

When the menacing Rottweiler family I fictionalised in 'Machete' moved out, a couple moved in with a kleptomaniac dog, Patch. Patch stole Ella's bowl, our little boy's sneakers, a bicycle spanner, a beach hat, any object we left on the veranda.

One day the local plumber, attending to our sewage line, saw Patch carrying off his conveniently bite-sized mobile phone. He couldn't catch him or retrieve his phone. Patch wasn't licensed and the plumber called the council dog-catcher. Our neighbour, who then had to bail out Patch from the pound, threatened to bash the plumber. 'I know where you live,' he said. The plumber told the police of the threat. They said they were keeping an eye on our neighbour, that he'd been in jail for robbery. Like his dog.

Ella, of course, fancied the canine thief and granted Patch rare liberties.

And then one day Patch, and his owner, were gone, having done a moonlight flit owing their landlord a month's rent.

Appropriately, it's a German, Volker Kriegel, whose shrewd and sardonic little book of dog cartoons, *Kriegels Kleine Hunde-Kunde* (*The Truth About Dogs*), perhaps gets closest today to capturing the abberant personalities of dogs: their essential vulgarity, gluttony, impudence, indiscretion, aggression, jealousy and silliness.

But his cartoons declare that dogs, for all their considerable faults, are what they are, and don't pretend otherwise. It's their owners who are devious, unpredictable, embarrassed and sentimental.

I don't buy that viewpoint a hundred per cent.

According to the well-known novelist Julian Barnes (*Flaubert's Parrot*), who translated Kriegel's book into English, the human race is distinctly fortunate that dogs have not yet learned how to blush.

The cartoonist and writer who brought bright fame to dogs was of course James Thurber, in the *New Yorker* and in his numerous books like *Men, Woman and Dogs*.

I think Thurber's sharp view of humans and his more accepting opinion of dogs is best shown in one famous cartoon. A man and dog hover fearfully on the edge of a forest on a wild and stormy night. The man gestures roughly

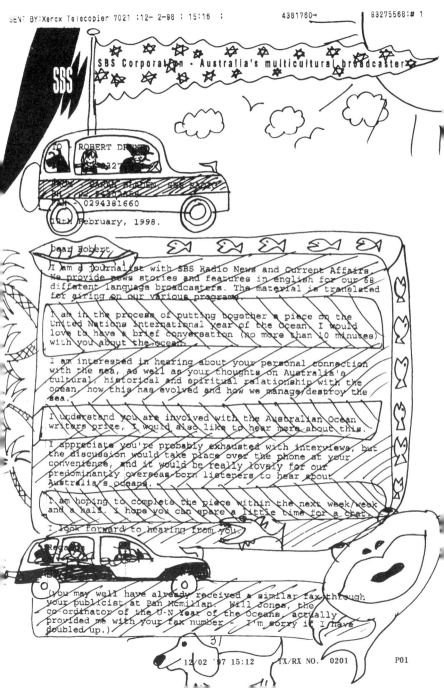

SBS Corporation - Australia's multicultural broadcaster

TO ROBERT DREWE
    327

FROM SARAH BLADEN SBS RADIO
PH - 02 9430 4268
FAX - 0294381660

12th February, 1998.

Dear Robert,

I am a journalist with SBS Radio News and Current Affairs.
We provide news stories and features in english for our 68
different language broadcasters. The material is translated
for airing on our various programs.

I am in the process of putting together a piece on the
United Nations International Year of the Ocean, I would
love to have a brief conversation (no more than 10 minutes)
with you about the ocean.

I am interested in hearing about your personal connection
with the sea, as well as your thoughts on Australia's
cultural, historical and spiritual relationship with the
ocean, how this has evolved and how we manage/destroy the
sea.

I understand you are involved with the Australian Ocean
writers prize, I would also like to hear more about this.

I appreciate you're probably exhausted with interviews, but
the discussion would take place over the phone at your
convenience, and it would be really lovely for our
predominantly overseas-born listeners to hear about
Australia's oceans.

I am hoping to complete the piece within the next week/week
and a half. I hope you can spare a little time for a chat.

I look forward to hearing from you.

Regards,

(you may well have already received a similar fax through
your publicist at Pan Mcmillan. Will Jones, the
co-ordinator of the U-N Year of the Oceans, actually
provided me with your fax number - I'm sorry if I have
doubled up.)

35

and shouts, 'Comb the woods!' The gentle dog, already turning back, looks up at him in disbelief.

The familiar Thurber dog first made his appearance in the collection of stories and illustrations, *The Seal in the Bedroom*. Thurber had always drawn dogs as a form of doodling while he was thinking, and as a practical joke on friends' and busy executives' memo pads, but now all the doodles became one dog, a serious, lop-eared fellow somewhere between a bloodhound and a basset hound, whose real-life model was the lithograph of the Duke of Westminster's hunting dogs hanging in his grandfather's hall. (When he started to draw them he found he hadn't left himself enough room to do the legs properly, so he shortened them.)

One of his childhood dogs, Muggs, was the original of 'The Dog That Bit People', and another, Rex, was the bull terrier memorialised in 'Snapshot of Rex'. When he was on the *New Yorker* staff, Thurber used to write letters home to Columbus, Ohio: 'Dear Father, Mother, Brother and Airedale.'

Muggs the Airedale 'always acted as if he thought he wasn't one of the family', although he didn't bite the family as often as he bit strangers. Thurber's mother insisted that it wasn't the dog's fault but the victims'. 'When he starts for them, they scream, and that excites him.'

Mrs Thurber used to make amends by sending Muggs's victims a box of candy every Christmas. This gesture became quite expensive. By the time Muggs died the list contained fifty names.

While Thurber's pathetic little husbands are constantly baffled or intimidated by cranky, overbearing wives, he allows them a special relationship with dogs. You can't help feeling for this desperate kind of kinship, given a tart, fanciful touch in one cartoon showing a man happily dancing with a very large dog.

The wife, meanwhile, disapproval etched in every line of her face and figure, says, 'Will you be good enough to dance this outside?'

Cartoonists love dogs because their position as put-upon domestic observers gives them the right to make ironic asides. The *New Yorker*'s dogs not only talk but also read, write, muse and have a superior insight into the absurdity of the human condition.

In one Peter Steiner cartoon, a dog sits obediently while a self-important little man addresses him thus: 'I've told you why I need a dog. Now suppose you tell me what makes you think you might be that dog.'

Complains an indignant hound in another Steiner cartoon: 'It's always "Sit", "Stay", "Heel", never "Think", "Innovate", "Be Yourself".'

As a compulsive lifetime doodler myself (dogs and fish mostly, plus the occasional hippo, cat and tycoon-with-cigar), I'm interested but not surprised that Thurber settled on a floppy-eared hound rather than a pointy-eared dog.

Hounds are more 'doodlable'. They don't take any emotional energy away from the doodler. If you doodle a pointy-eared dog you right away start thinking about teeth and a snarling expression. You're soon thinking about adding one of those tough, spike-studded dog collars. Next thing you're doing a *drawing*. Rather than just doodling, you're involved in the project. The dog-drawing has become more important than the telephone conversation or thought process it was supposed to be complementing. The pointy-eared dog has become the point.

The true doodle, however, can be, and should be, left half-finished when the primary activity or thought is over. (Or easily turned into a skyscraper or ocean liner.) Anyway, when you draw a hound the ears and jowls say it all. You can forget about their legs. This is just as well, because the rear legs – the way they bend backwards from a sort of reverse knee arrangement – are hard to draw and never convincing.

Interestingly, most famous cartoon dogs have been floppy-eared. Think of Disney's Pluto, Charles Schulz's Snoopy and MGM's Droopy. Also Fred Basset. The only people who doodle German shepherds are the owners of German shepherds. And they never stop. There's one in every office, just as there is at least one young woman who constantly doodles horses.

What's the matter with German-shepherd owners? They're the ones who introduced those sad, defensive bumper-stickers declaring their love for their choice of dog breed. Doberman, bull terrier and Rottweiler owners jumped in next. What can I say? Shorthaired-pointer owners have no need – or wish – to declare their choice of pet to the nation's motorists.

There is a definite park protocol for saying hello.

Before 7.30 a.m. there is greater camaraderie between individual dog-walking strangers. It's OK then, almost compulsory, to say good morning. (But only if he or she, like you, has a dog in tow.) There is a hearty feeling that both of you are in this early-morning activity together, and are maybe even a little intrepid.

After 8 a.m. the friendliness dwindles to a nod. The nod gets curter as the day progresses. Speaking is out, unless you both have the same breed of dog, of course, in which case you're members of the same club, like MG drivers, and are welcome to speak freely at any hour, comparing their habits, misadventures and dire effects on your lives. (That last category is usually initiated by me.)

The same freedom applies when one of you is walking a very small puppy. Then it's acceptable to stop and pat the puppy, chortle at its antics and, if the puppy-owner initiates it, respond to a friendly conversational overture.

Saying hello in the park after sunset is not done. No one who isn't a same-breed owner or puppy owner and/or a cruising homosexual says hello at or after dusk.

Mind you, the hearty greeting of ambulant strangers can be quite tedious and exhausting, as anyone walking in England's Lake District, home of the compulsory early-morning hello (and last haunt of hikers in tweed plus-fours), can attest.

Professional dog-walkers work the park every day – Jan, Jane, Robyn and five or six others. They wear Akubra hats and R.M. Williams boots, and are tanned from life in the open air. Their belts jangle with the keys of many valuable Eastern Suburbs houses.

Some of them exercise ten or twelve dogs at a time, whirling and crashing through the muddy pampas grass of the park's

Murder Across the River

Blood River.

This Side of the River

The Murder Side of the River

Swimming in the Black River

north end with their roistering packs of canines – from little puffballs to semi-wolves.

In emergencies we've called on their services. Ella would always run away from Robyn, tear across six lanes of major road and, after a few snacks en route, arrive home, whining. Poor Robyn, after desperate searches in the surrounding streets, had to expel her from her dog club.

Ella the loner didn't fancy the shared experienced. But she will usually stay obedient with Jane, perhaps because she walks only one other dog at a time. This is Bert, a mad Irish setter. He's a shambling, slobbering idiot, owned by a Bellevue Hill judge with no time to walk him. Ella and Bert like each other's style.

Ella works on the old kids' rule of dogs: floppy ears means stupid, pointy ears means bite. Needless to say she likes the stupid ones. While she'll go a long way to avoid German shepherds and cattle dogs, setters and hounds have her approval. She seems to instinctively recognise other shorthaired pointers. The more a dog looks like her, the better she likes it.

She likes women more than men as a rule. Outside the family she likes her holiday minder, Jan, most of all.

The other day a dog-walker was having trouble coaxing one of his clients into his van. The dog was lying just out of reach, chewing a pine cone.

The man said crossly: 'Spike, you're too old for that crap and so am I!'

———————————

The professional dog-walkers' beat is much the same as the park's gay beat. Both groups cruise the paths through the northern, wooded, Oxford Street end. The only difference is that the dog-walkers usually eventually congregate in the open field below, by the commemoration building.

A mob of dogs will suddenly tumble out of the bushes and crash past a lone, bare-torsoed man posing and flexing in his G-string on a rock or tree stump. Apart from a momentary lapse of poise, no harm is done.

This happens more often in warm weather. If the dog-walkers suspect they might be about to interrupt something in the bushes, they give due warning by raising the noise level, calling and whistling the dogs. Occasionally, of course, the dogs crash right through.

The only people I've seen openly fornicating in the park were a heterosexual couple lying on the path beside a pond at high noon one sunny Sunday. They were oblivious to the sun, the hour, the pedestrian traffic. Ella gave them a good sniff as we passed.

But who knows what human and animal activities happen in the total privacy of those round, bushy palms, resembling leafy igloos or African huts, which separate the ponds from the horse exercise area? I've seen derelicts crawling from them in the mornings after a night's sleep, and sheepish high-school lovers, buttoning up their uniforms and removing twigs from their hair, emerging on Wednesday sports afternoons. And of course the possums scampering out at dusk.

One of Ella's more common and sordid park discoveries is the used condom. There's a special sort of grim, slapstick embarrassment in watching – or trying to avoid watching – her proud and vigorous display of a condom.

As she swings it around in her teeth, an activity she feels bound to do as close as possible to complete strangers, some mysterious vibration gathers an instant audience of toddlers, mothers, fathers – and especially grandmothers – and my curious son.

While every adult tries their damnedest to stay cool ('Yes, darling, the doggy found a balloon. Shall we go and have an icecream now?'), the tension runs from face to face like a Mexican wave. Fathers have a particular tight smile for each other on these occasions.

But you don't need to be a grandma or in the company of small children to find the used condom and the discarded syringe the most confronting, mood-destroying and depressing examples of modern public detritus.

———————————

One night on the Central Coast, Ella and her kleptomaniac friend Patch from next door chased our cat, Boots, onto the roof. The small black cat sat up there in the moonlight, clearly defined on the silver iron roof.

Boots was spotted up there by a Powerful Owl, a big species of owl known in the coastal hills for living on possums and squirrel-gliders. We had seen the owl a few nights before, perched on our window-sill. We had felt eyes on us and sensed we were being spied on. We looked up suddenly and saw this big grey and white owl, nearly a metre high, peering in at us, sizing up the situation.

Boots was the size of a possum. Suddenly there was a swift, flurried bang on the roof and the cat was gone. Boots was killed by an owl, but Ella and her friend were responsible for chasing her up on the roof and making her an easy target.

If the principals in this slaughter were humans Ella would be facing a manslaughter rap.

This owl and pussycat story demonstrates the dilemma of using a real pet incident in fiction.

A female writer used this occurrence as the basis for a short story about a couple with a new baby whose cat is taken from their roof by an owl. The wife had been too exhausted from new motherhood to lift the crying cat down. Anyway this was usually the man's job. (The man, of course, was blissfully asleep. Not that this lets him off the hook.)

The woman in the story suffers deep guilt for the cat's death, and deepened resentment towards her sleeping husband for a recent, but terminated, adulterous love affair he has had.

In real life the husband hadn't had any such extra-marital affair and, reading the manuscript before publication, was miffed that this angle, for whatever reason, had been introduced into an otherwise realistic story. In fact she had given it a twist. Some dialogue she had given her female character was dialogue he himself had expressed in the past.

In real life the only sin he was guilty of was snoring through the real cat's misadventure on the roof.

The story was published as the title piece in a collection of short stories. Of course they had told all their friends of the owl swooping off with their cat. Everyone knew this, just as they knew the couple had a new baby. So, reading it, they believed the remainder of the story, too. (Writers know that inserting even one fact into a piece of fiction gives the whole thing veracity.)

The woman's story had the main female character becoming sadder but shrewder at the end. Wiser. An owl even. The real-life man, on the other hand, came out of the whole business feeling like a pussycat who'd been chased onto the roof.

Ella sniffed around for the cat for a few days but she didn't miss it at all.

When our city landlord announces one of his lightning visits we guiltily hide all traces of Ella. Our lease discourages pets. That means vacuuming the floors and sofa, hiding her food and water bowls, her leads and all her chewy things.

I'm eliminating all Ella evidence from the back yard. Watching myself hosing her turds in the garden, trying to break them down with a strong jet of water, I feel pathetic and desperate. And nauseated.

I hide her bed under the house. In doing so I discover a huge new hole she has dug there. It must be two metres deep. All sorts of pipes and wires are exposed, and the sides of the house's foundations.

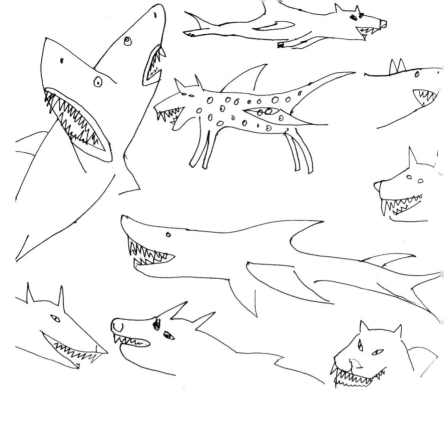

I urgently place a plastic wading pool over the hole. Then I take Ella for a walk, and keep her in the back of the car, parked in the street, until the landlord has gone.

It's then I notice that her favourite dog toys – the red rubber chicken drumstick and yellow rubber hamburger – have been lying on the veranda throughout his visit.

One afternoon in a wooded area of the park I have the eerie feeling of being watched. I turn around and a wolf is standing on a rocky outcrop above me, lone and quiet, staring down at me.

Its ears are pointed high on its head, its eyes are slanted. Except they're pale blue. It turns out to be a male husky. Its owner says that after several generations in Australia his branch of the breed has adapted to the heat and grown a thinner coat, no thicker than a German shepherd's. When she took him down to the south coast one winter his coat grew thick again.

What about his strange proud wolflike demeanour? 'He likes to stand on a high spot and survey things, get the lie of the land,' she says.

Of course Ella is nowhere to be seen. At first glimpse and sniff of the wolfish dog she has dematerialised.

Consider the quandary of two people heading towards each other on the same narrow path: when to give way?

It's usually when they're about twenty metres apart that they step aside. Earlier than that and they look over-polite or paranoid. Any later and closer than that and the situation can seem a touch weird and aggressive.

But once they've spotted each other you know the only thing on each mind is: when will I step aside?

There's a narrow path on the top of a knoll at the south end of the park. When two normally polite people approach each other on this path there's a funny scene where they're both toddling obliquely along the side of the hill while the flat, empty, walkable path yawns between them.

Of course when one of the people in a path confrontation is a serious jogger there is a protocol that the (more serene) walker gives way. Just the opposite to the old water give-way rule of Sail before Steam.

———————

This morning Ella barks at a bearded woman in the park. The woman's reaction totally bamboozles her. The woman bares her own teeth like a dog, shakes up the can of Coke she is carrying and squirts it at Ella.

Ella runs off, sticky and bewildered. The woman takes a defiant swig from her can and strides on.

Genetically inclined to notice and chase a flapping, stumbling, wounded animal, Ella can't resist barking at and bounding after any creature she thinks is out of the ordinary. She has an extremely sensitive antenna to abnormality. Any body-language that's unusual, boisterous or over-tentative excites her.

This is unerringly politically-incorrect, as well as infuriating and frightening to people with limps, walking frames, umbrellas, rustling plastic bags, jerky walking styles, booming voices, flowing garments, timid movements (anyone with a cultural mistrust of dogs, like many Asians). And beards.

Embarrassingly, people who are physically or mentally disabled are top of her list. She also hates drunks and show-offs who lurch and prod at her. She dislikes angry men, men in snappy hats, people with scarves wound around their faces, people dressed in rags, hippies, people who are stoned, and gushy women.

She ignores people who ignore her. The same goes for dogs not on leads. She will bark bravely at any dog on a lead or safely behind a fence. She will chase a cat as long as it runs away. Any cat that stands its ground she pretends not to notice. Then she nonchalantly crosses the road to avoid it.

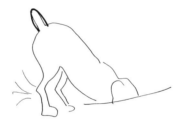

Adjectives to describe Ella: Insolent. Sometimes abject. Affectionate at times. But her affection is of the toadying, prison-trustee variety: What's in it for me? The old lag in charge of the jail library. The insincere petty thief who makes the warders' tea.

When she walks she undulates, wagging her bottom like a streetwalker or a racehorse. She also varies between

acceptably lean and sinewy (all her ribs should be
showing, according to *The German Shorthaired Pointer*)
and a barrel on legs, depending on whether she has recently
escaped from custody and wolfed down the contents of
the street's garbage bins.

She deliberately loses her licence tag, name and address.
She's scared of umbrellas, hockey sticks, cricket bats, brave
cats, paper bags, balloons, whoopee cushions and men
outside pubs. Turn your back for a second and she's gone.

She can also flap her ears so they crack like a whip.

The heat from her body can dry socks. (She sleeps in
the laundry.)

The German Shorthaired Pointer, however, sees her thus:
'An aristocratic, well-balanced, symmetrical animal with
conformation indicating power, endurance and agility and
a look of intelligence and animation. The first impression
is of a keenness which denotes full enthusiasm for work
without indication of nervous or flighty character. Grace
of outline, clean-cut head, sloping shoulders, deep chest,
powerful back, strong quarters, good bone composition,
adequate muscle, well-carried tail and taut coat all combine
to produce a look of nobility.'

She has only once caught another creature. This was an
already wounded coot. She carried it self-consciously around

in her mouth for an hour (having been bred to do so) until she either sucked it to death or it had a heart attack.

In all fairness, it must be said that Ella, when in the mood and indoors, is a good sport. She'll put up with all sorts of indignities for a game.

Firmly directed by the youngest boy, she has played the part of a cow, a wolf, a fox, a hyena, a lion, a horse, a dog-fish, a crocodile and a shark. Also a nun, a pirate chief and – her most testing role – an old peasant woman who is actually Snow White's evil stepmother, the Queen, in disguise.

She's the kind of dog a child feels compelled to dress up. Indoors, she'll wear a headscarf and sunglasses without looking too depressed. I think she secretly enjoys being covered. A towel reminds her of being dried after a bath, and sends her whirling round in frenzied circles, but a blanket is quite calming. Until you remove the blanket she'll lie 'doggo' and completely hidden. If you forget, that's fine. Even with very little air she manages to have a nice snooze or, rather, trance.

The small boy has a favourite game called 'Africa'. The point of 'Africa' is for him and me – the 'explorers' – to run down the corridor from one bedroom to another, holding hands, with a 'lion' hot on our heels.

Because the lion is actually much faster than the perpetually terrified explorers, there's a lot of yelling in the game of 'Africa'. If they do safely reach 'Africa' (the parents' bed), however, the explorers can't just rest around the campfire. They must pull their legs up sharply, yelling a lot, so their dangling feet don't suddenly tempt the 'crocodile'.

'Africa' is a game that may be played for seconds or hours, depending on whether one of the explorers gets over-stimulated and has a crying fit before bed and whether the lion/crocodile gets bored with the sameness of the chase and saunters downstairs to the sofa.

———————————

Visiting the real Africa, Zimbabwe and Zambia, while researching *The Drowner* brings home just how important the territorial imperative is to animals. It's an eye-opener to me. Everyone knows territory is a major impulse but I hadn't realised the extent to which it occupies animals' time.

It seems to come well before food, reproduction and shelter in their priorities. The spraying, scratching, secreting, urinating and building of dung middens never ceases. Life is all about endlessly, relentlessly, leaving your mark. Building a fence. Staking a claim. Suddenly you begin to understand the urban graffiti of the dispossessed, the carved initials on the school desk, the compulsive suburban trimmer of next door's overhanging branches.

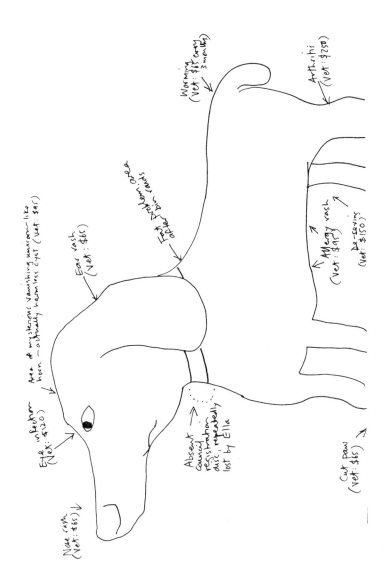

Worming
(Vet: $15 every
3 months)

Arthritis
(Vet: $250)

Area of mysterious vanishing unicorn-like
horn — actually harmless cyst (Vet: $45)

Empty Problem area
after big walks

Ear rash
(Vet: $65)

Allergy rash
(Vet: $95)

De-sexing
(Vet: $150)

Eye infection
(Vet: $120)

Nose rash
(Vet: $65)

Absent →
council
registration
disc, repeatedly
lost by Ella

Cut Paw
(Vet: $65)

It certainly puts Ella's nightly before-bed, bladder-emptying walk around the block in perspective. Waiting on street corners at midnight for her to go, it had always annoyed me that she would hold on, even though I knew she'd gulped down a whole bowl of water hours before and that her bladder was full.

The way I saw it, if creatures needed to go they went. I didn't realise the extent that dogs saved it. Ella actually *harnesses* it. She *marshals* her urine resources. Like every dog, she sniffs around until she finds another dog's markings, and then expends sufficient urine to obliterate its mark, to say, 'This is Ella's territory and (literally) piss off.'

But she won't squirt a skerrick more than necessary. She won't urinate indiscriminately. She can (and how painful a human would find this!) abruptly stop and hold it in again until another thimbleful is needed. In an inner-city suburb with a dog in most households, this can be amazingly often or infuriatingly seldom.

The sites present no problems. Any bitch can do it on the grass; Ella can do it on the sides of garbage bins, telegraph poles, trees. A most liberated female, she can piss like a male. She can raise a leg. And – just to confuse next-door's Rottweiler – to a respectable height.

She can go ten times in the length of a block, or not at all. The last walk of the day can take some time.

———————————

How to put this delicately? From behind, Ella is sometimes mistaken for a male. When this happens the person who has made the error is slightly embarrassed and mutters apologies. And I'm vaguely embarrassed, too, on Ella's behalf.

Her vulva is big, sways when she walks and in its divided roundness has a similarity to testes.

The German Shorthaired Pointer, discussing show standards, says sternly, 'Doggy bitches and bitchy dogs are to be faulted.' I feel I must whisper this. *Is Ella in fact a doggy bitch?*

She knows who she is, however, and no one better mess with her around that area! She's not having any of that nonsense.

Why do I almost feel as if I've betrayed a confidence in writing this?

———————————

I wonder whether bitches know when they've been spayed. Do they think they're 'missing out'? The vet says of course not and gives me a funny look. The canine behaviourists say maybe.

Favorite foods:

1. Chicken (fried)
2. Barbecue leftovers
3. Corpses
4. Asian
5. Indefinable garbage
6. Bread for the ducks
7. Chum.
8. Pal
9. Apple cores
10. Manure

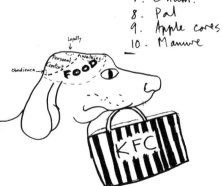

Ella had her 'operation' at six months. Her spaying didn't appear to set her back a jot. It made no difference to her vigour or her appetite. Even my daughters, more sentimental than I am, agree Ella isn't the maternal type.

She certainly has a *je ne regrette rien* attitude. She doesn't much like puppies. She gets all middle-aged and disapproving when they're around. She's a bit of a loner. In the park she still avoids most of her old contemporaries in the dog-walking teams. She will walk around the outskirts of an area to avoid a strange dog. She hates German shepherds and is frightened of them, having once been set upon by a pair of them. Her favourite dogs are boisterous but unthreatening males (no funny business, thanks) her own size and age.

We don't regret the absence of oestrus either. *The German Shorthaired Pointer* carries advertisements for 'Anne Ardmore's Doggie Pads ("Sanitary Pads for Female Dogs in Season") and Doggie Britches ("The Modern Sanitary Garment")'. They come in pink packets with an illustration of a saucy, be-padded or pantied poodle on the front.

At the stage of having to buy and administer Anne Ardmore's Doggie Britches, I think dogs and I would permanently part company.

Speaking of African animals, the white-hunter culture (*pace* Wilbur Smith's novels) insists that, in conversation, plural animals should be referred to in the singular, as in six lion, four elephant, two rhino, five giraffe, etc.

To say, 'Look at all the zebras!' invites the smug response, 'Yes, I'd say there were over a hundred *zebra* there.'

Outside Africa this odd principle mostly relates (just as weirdly) to grass-eating creatures with hoofs. (Buffalo, bison, deer, sheep, elk, antelope, and so on.) In Africa, where the trees are surprisingly full of monkey and the rivers swarm with hippo and crocodile, the habit is all-encompassing.

As I said to our boring ex-Rhodesian safari-guide, 'I can't wait to get home to my three dog.' I don't have that many, thank God, but he was making my nerves jangle.

The habit has the same grating effect on me as pretentious people referring to films or movies as *film* or, worse, *cinema*. When did people stop saying they were 'going to the pictures'? When did this singular nonsense start? With film reviewers? Books will be next. They'll be saying, 'Have you read any good *library* lately?'

———

A pertinent item in today's *Herald*: 'In the latest *Australian Family Physician*, Dr Amanda Shue describes being called to a house where she found a naked, dead woman in the bathroom with one nipple and other body parts missing.

The shower was running and the doctor's first thoughts were of a psychotic killer. But a subsequent autopsy revealed that the woman had died from an asthma attack.

"The fact that the family labrador had done away with loyalties and had tucked in was confirmed when he was put down and the grisly evidence found in his stomach," says Dr Shue.

The experience had taught her that asthma is still a potentially fatal disease and that dogs are only masquerading as domestic pets.'

German dogs are usually exceptionally, well, German. They look as if they could lead Panzer divisions, or at least follow them. Think of German shepherds, Dobermans, schnauzers, Rottweilers. Don't they look German? Even those pale-furred, blue-eyed Weimaraners.

But not German shorthaired pointers. They're definitely civilians: good-looking, sleek, Mediterranean layabouts – casual and disorderly. Pointy-headed shirkers, more like it. If they were humans they'd always be out at nightclubs and calling in sick next day.

Of course no dog is more suited to the discipline and punishment professions than the German shepherd.

However, they do have a couple of vulnerable areas: the hips and feet. Fortunately, these weaknesses have recently been bolstered by the invention of dog boots.

The boots were specially designed for Britain's prison and police dogs, who can cut their paws on glass and debris in the course of their work quelling human disturbances. The boots have rubber soles lined with an aluminium-armoured layer, followed by cushioned material under the dog's paw. In appearance like miniature Doc Martens' boots, they fasten with either laces or Velcro and come in eighteen sizes. Each dog wears two different pairs, with a bigger size for the larger front paws.

They look extremely silly but, according to Steven Allen, governor of Britain's prison dogs, 'Wearing boots makes no difference to the German shepherds' performance and they soon seem to forget they're wearing them.'

Other working-dog agencies are very enthusiastic about the boots. Search dogs who have to get in amongst sharp rubble will soon be wearing them. And in New Mexico, where German shepherds are used in border patrols, their paws need protection from the hot sand when they're rounding up Mexicans.

Today Ella runs gleefully through the park, scandalising mothers and children, with the head of a Sacred Ibis in her mouth.

The ibis's head has been separated from its body, presumably (from the smell) by a much earlier dog. She's holding it by its long, hooked beak so it looks like she's carrying an umbrella handle.

It really stinks. When she is far enough away from me she drops it and performs a shoulder roll on it, then picks it up again as I approach and runs off.

There are plenty more ibises where that came from. The islands in the park's lakes swarm with them. They are even driving out the swans and swamp hens. At sunset the ibises fly home in majestic V formation to their squatters' islands after a busy day ransacking the bins of Darlinghurst.

The streetwise ibis is an odd sight – that long, narrow beak piercing and protruding through a styrofoam Big Mac container – especially if you associate the bird with a dignified ancient backdrop and Egyptian hieroglyphics.

When did they suddenly appear in central Sydney, taking over the scavenger role from pigeons and seagulls? I can't remember a single ibis around five years ago.

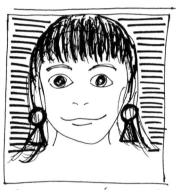

The people who like her most

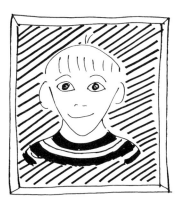

63

At six months Ella celebrated her grown-up teeth by dragging a dead pelican out of the lake and eating it. It took her three visits to the park but she managed to consume it – beak, feathers and all.

When I'd attempt to extract her from the carcass she'd run away with it, of course. Hidden inside it, she'd bolt down the path, the wind catching its feathers. This stinking apparition, with its six-foot wingspan and huge lolling beak, made quite an impression galloping through the toddlers' playground.

She couldn't be put off her ludicrous and distasteful task. This relentless panache reminded me of those European performers who for some reason feel driven to slowly eat bicycles or to render down grandfather clocks with their teeth.

With the same determined, self-important frown (someone has to do it!) she dispatches today a very dead fox she discovers up at the coast. It's so stiff when she finds it that she's able to carry it proudly around all day, holding it in front of her by the tip of its tail.

This flag-bearing display is a disconcertingly cannibalistic as well as grisly sight. The fox, thus attenuated by rigor mortis, is a fair bit longer than she is. And she knows it. For a whole morning she struts about boasting and pretending that she's killed it. Then she munches it all up, from nose-tip to tail-tip.

Not counting road-killed cats which she enjoys, the flatter, older and thinner (family-sized pizza shape), the better, the fox is possibly the first carnivore she's eaten. Her primary cadaver diet is decayed possums, swamp hens and rabbits and, on the coast, dead cormorants, gulls and old fishermen's bait. (Ancient prawns and octopus tentacles are a delicacy.) When the park rangers occasionally cull the numbers of giant carp from the ponds, she does enjoy a bloated, several-days-out-of-the-water carp or two.

Her tastes, however, are as catholic as nature allows. They range from the faeces of any species (from terriers to park tramps) to random bites of lavender, freesias and pine cones. But, alas for breath-sweetening possibilities, not necessarily in that order.

By far the smallest animals she has consumed – a sad day – would have to be the several hundred sea-monkeys she drank when my son left their jar unattended on the floor.

At the park she likes to finish off her meal (perhaps some burnt barbecue sausages from the garbage bin, following a starter of horse manure) with a muddy swim and a hearty draught from a pond. They all carry warning signs saying *Danger – Blue-green Algae, Keep Dogs Away*, but try telling her that.

At what age do we humans learn to be disgusted? It's surely a learned process. The way young children's minds frame the world in many cases isn't all that different from dogs' behaviour.

The MIT psychologist Dr Steven Pinker's popular treatise, *How the Mind Works*, relays with relish his findings that 62 per cent of toddlers were prepared to eat fake dog faeces (made of peanut butter and smelly cheese), believing it to be the real thing.

The German Shorthaired Pointer: 'The breed as a whole possesses very great scenting ability. On wounded game the shorthair knows no peer. As surely as his keen nose can pick the body scent of game from the air, he can put his head down and track rapidly-moving crippled fur or feather and bring it back to hand.'

––––––––––––––––

Her dietary habits, especially her preference for the murky, smelly, allegedly dangerous pond-water over the ordinary tap water supplied for dogs, suggest a book to me. (She has also tried poisonous snail-killing pellets, but apart from some exotic green droppings, appeared none the worse for the experience.)

I toy with the idea of writing a children's story called 'The Toxic Dog'. Then the title suddenly brings to mind Henry Lawson's famous story 'The Loaded Dog'.

Now I consider updating or reworking the Lawson story. As I walk through the park I get the usual rush of enthusiasm that comes with a new idea.

So I look up 'The Loaded Dog' and, greatly impressed by the laudatory quotation from Joseph Conrad on the jacket of *The Penguin Henry Lawson* ('Lawson's sketches are beyond praise'), check to see if it resonates more than thirty years since I last read it – and one hundred years since he wrote it.

Lawson's story, last studied in Mr Altofer's ninth-grade English class, is famous for its comedy and for the harsh 'bushman's' treatment of its canine characters.

Lawson sentimentally anthropomorphises his dogs, ascribing good and evil personalities to them. But when he dispatches them he does so with a relish that would unsettle Walt Disney, much less the RSPCA.

The humour of 'The Loaded Dog' centres on the actions of the dog in question, the idiotic black retriever, Tommy. Academics have argued that Lawson cleverly edges the story away from stock farce by making what happens the result of his master, Dave Regan's, bright idea to construct an elaborate blasting-powder cartridge to bomb the fish out of a waterhole.

It still looks like stock farce to me. Lawson scholars obviously never see any early-morning TV cartoons.

With a couple of quid-each-way touches at the end, Lawson abrogates responsibility for the story and turns it into another of his Dave Regan yarns, another outback campfire myth. Lawson scholars think this was deft of him; I think the story is trivialised by three or four unnecessary final paragraphs. A soft populist touch.

Lawson's Tommy of course snatches up the lighted, spluttering cartridge in his slobbering, grinning mouth – and then tries to return it to his masters, Dave, Jim Bently and Andy Page, who flee in panic and try to hide in a nearby shanty pub. There, under the kitchen, lurks a 'vicious yellow mongrel cattle-dog sulking and nursing his nastiness'. This dog, Lawson writes, is 'a sneaking, fighting, thieving canine whom neighbours had tried for years to shoot or poison'.

Anyway, the nasty yellow dog chases and bites the foolish but friendly retriever, who drops the cartridge and runs off. The cattle-dog goes back to see what it is that Tommy's dropped. A dozen or so of his pack follow him: 'spidery, thievish, cold-blooded kangaroo dogs, mongrel sheep- and cattle-dogs, vicious black and yellow dogs – that slip after you in the dark, nip your heels, and vanish without explaining – and yapping, yelping small fry'.

The nasty yellow dog sniffs at the cartridge twice, and is just taking a third cautious sniff when . . .

Then follows the only sentence in the story which was worth a second look by the coarse and bloodthirsty fourteen-year-olds of Mr Altofer's English class:

'When the smoke and dust cleared away, the remains of the nasty yellow dog were lying against the paling fence of the yard looking as if he had been kicked into a fire by a horse and afterwards rolled in the dust under a barrow, and finally thrown against the fence from a distance.'

'The Loaded Dog' still seems a juvenile yarn. Not for the first time I'm disappointed in Lawson – and in myself for failing to appreciate his mythical status in Australian literature.

The bush culture – and the Australian education system of the past – didn't encourage the mollycoddling of dogs.

For the first sixty years of the twentieth century children in most states were taught to read from the eight-volume Victorian Readers. The learning-to-read experience that stands out in the minds of most Australians over forty is the story 'The Hobyahs' from the second book of the Victorian Readers.

Intended for six-year-olds, 'The Hobyahs' (author unknown) goes like this:

> *Once upon a time, a little old woman and a little old man lived in the bush in a hut all made of bark. They had a little yellow dog called Dingo. The little yellow dog always barked when any one came near the hut. (Real dingoes do not bark – they howl; but this dog barked.)*
>
> *One night, when the little old woman and the little old man were fast asleep, out from the gloomy gullies came the hobyahs, creep, creep, creeping.*
>
> *Through the grey gum-trees came the hobyahs, run, run, running.*
>
> *Skip, skip, skipping on the ends of their toes ran the hobyahs.*
>
> *And the hobyahs cried, 'Pull down the hut, eat up the little old man, carry off the little old woman.'*
>
> *Then yellow dog Dingo ran out, barking loudly. The hobyahs were afraid. They ran home as fast as they could go.*
>
> *But the little old man woke up from his dream and cried, 'Little dog Dingo barks so loud that I can neither slumber nor sleep. In the morning I will take off his tail.' So the little old man took off little dog Dingo's tail to stop him from barking.*

A tragic tale of Greed

A few years ago, a client called us to relay some sad news about Gerta, her 3-year-old Spaniel mix. It seemed that while her owner was out of the house, Gerta got into a large box of chocolates that had been left out on the coffee table the night before. Chocolate is tempting to dogs because it contains dairy products, sugar, and various oils. Unfortunately, it also contains the chemical *theobromine*, a substance that is extremely toxic to dogs. Gerta scented out the chocolates and proceeded to eat the entire box. Weighing in at only 15 or 20 pounds, the few pounds of chocolate she consumed was enough to prove lethal.

This sad story illustrates how important it is to make the home a safe place for Bobo to live in. Just as you "baby-proof" your home and property to safeguard your child, so must you "dog-proof" your pet's territory to prevent physical or psychological trauma from occurring. Although some dogs never show an interest in potentially dangerous items around the home, most do at some time or other. You must deal with this possibility.

Solution: Safeguard Bobo's Environment

Dogs are curious by nature and are driven to investigate every nook and cranny of their environment. Their excellent sense of smell plays a pivotal role in this function. If an interesting smell wafts out from a kitchen cabinet, rest assured little Bobo will want to go in there and check it out. When he does, he will discover many potentially toxic items. The garbage, probably his first target, may contain dangerous items such as chicken bones, broken glass, sharp lids from open cans, food packaging that Bobo could choke on. At the least, he could end up eating discarded food and getting a bad case of diarrhea.

The garbage, however, is probably the least dangerous item that Bobo could get into, under the kitchen sink. Most people also keep a myriad of chemicals here, including ammonia- and bleach-based cleaners, detergents, drain cleaner, furniture polish, house plant

The second night, along came the hobyahs. Out from the gloomy gullies came the hobyahs, creep, creep, creeping.

Through the grey gum-trees came the hobyahs, run, run, running.

Skip, skip, skipping on the ends of their toes, ran the hobyahs.

And the hobyahs cried, 'Pull down the hut, eat up the little old man, carry off the little old woman.'

The yellow dog Dingo ran out, barking loudly. The hobyahs were afraid. They ran home as fast as they could go.

But the little old man tossed in his sleep and cried, 'Little dog Dingo barks so loud that I can neither slumber nor sleep. In the morning I will take off his legs.' So the little old man took off little dog Dingo's legs to stop him from barking.

The third night along came the hobyahs. Out from the gloomy gullies came the hobyahs, creep, creep, creeping.

Through the grey gum-trees came the hobyahs, run, run, running.

Skip, skip, skipping on the ends of their toes, ran the hobyahs.

And the hobyahs cried, 'Pull down the hut, eat up the little old man, carry off the little old woman.'

The yellow dog Dingo ran out, barking loudly. The hobyahs were afraid. They ran home as fast as they could go.

But the little old man heard Dingo. He sat up in bed and cried, 'Little dog Dingo barks so loud that I can neither slumber nor sleep. In the morning I will take off his head.' So the little old man took off Dingo's head. Then the little dog Dingo could not bark any more.

That night along came the hobyahs.

Through the long grass came the hobyahs, creep, creep, creeping.

Through the grey gum-trees came the hobyahs, run, run, running.

Skip, skip, skipping on the ends of their toes, ran the hobyahs.

And the hobyahs cried, 'Pull down the hut, eat up the little old man, carry off the little old woman.'

Now the little dog Dingo could not bark any more. There was no one to frighten the hobyahs away.

They pulled down the hut. They took the little old woman away in their bag. But the little old man they could not get, for he hid himself under the bed.

Then the hobyahs went home. They hung the bag upon a big hook. In it was the little old woman.

They poked the bag with their fingers and cried, 'Ha! ha! little old woman.'

But when the sun came up they went to sleep. Hobyahs, you know, used to sleep all day.

When the little old man found the little old woman was gone, he was very sorry.

Now he knew what a good little dog Dingo had been.

So he took Dingo's tail and his legs and his head and gave them back to him.

Then little dog Dingo went sniffing and sniffing along to find the little old woman.

Soon he came to the hobyahs' house. He heard the little old woman crying in the bag.

He saw that the hobyahs were all fast asleep.

Then he cut open the bag with his sharp teeth.

Out jumped the little old woman, and ran home again as fast as she could go.

Dingo did not run away, but crept inside the bag to hide.

When night came, the hobyahs woke up, and they poked it with their long fingers.

They cried, 'Ha! ha! little old woman.'

*Out of the bag jumped little dog Dingo, and ate up every
one of the hobyahs.*

And that is why there are no hobyahs now.

A woman friend, a well-known novelist, told me recently
she was still having nightmares about the hobyahs forty-five
years after primary school. I was glad to hear this because
variations on the hobyahs, some tribe or platoon of
mysterious unspecified enemies, invade my dreams about
once a week.

I think Jung would have plenty to say about the hobyahs.
Perhaps after all these years they're embedded in the
collective unconscious of the nation.

Indeed, I wonder whether it's the ingrained fear of hobyahs
in Australians over forty that has given rise to some recent
unseemly political movements and government decisions.

———————————

Dogs are usually treated with cloying sentimentality in
books and films. Think about Steinbeck's dog in *Travels
with Charlie*. What a disappointingly lovable, loyal and floppy
Nobel Prize-winner's dog he turned out to be.

As a child of three or four I loved *The Poky Little Puppy* in
the well-known Golden Books series. He's a naughty hound

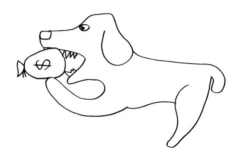

pup (remarkably like a shorthaired pointer) who escapes each day by digging a hole under the fence against his mother's instructions, comes home late every night and eats everyone else's pudding.

My little boy has the book, too. It's now a classic. *The Poky Little Puppy* has a catchy, repetitive rhythm and a cheeky central character for children to identify with. It has never been out of print since being published in 1942.

As an author I can only deeply sympathise with its creator, Janette Sebring Lowrey, and illustrator, Gustaf Tenngren, and their descendants. Golden Books (over one billion books sold) pays its authors an upfront sum, so they've missed out on sixty-four years' worth of royalties so far.

———————————

My youngest son loves those live-action films about heroic labradors and golden retrievers who walk unerringly across North America in search of their owners who have moved house after death or divorce.

After ferocious fights with mountain lions, humorous brushes with porcupines and skunks and incredible feats of mountain-climbing and lake-fording endurance this sort of dog finds his way to the very Vancouver or Seattle suburban street and sunset-burnished bungalow where his twelve-year-old master is sadly kicking at autumn leaves and pining for him.

Sometimes a heroic dog will accomplish this uncanny journey from the East Coast, say, in uneasy partnership with a cat – in which case the cat, although anti-heroic and a sarcastic smart-arse (and, if a male, possessing sibilant, stereotypical homosexual speech), will at some crucial stage save the dog's life.

Classics of the genre are *Benji*, *Homeward Bound* and *The Incredible Journey*. Their canine characters differ from their heroic movie ancestors Rin Tin Tin, Stronghart and Lassie in that they're not known – before their particular adventures, at least – to be particularly brave. They're shopping-mall versions of Old Yeller, just ordinary suburban pets whose devotion and internal radar prevail against the great odds of the wilderness.

Just as I tried to will my droopy Shep into a hero many years ago, my son fervently wishes Ella was this brave stamp of a dog.

———————————

I remember first seeing *Rin Tin Tin* in the Baptist church hall in Waratah Avenue as an eight-year-old. The Baptists were on a school-holiday recruiting drive and screened blurry ancient silent movies in an attempt to win us over. After Rinty we had to sit and sing 'Jesus Wants Me For A Sunbeam' and the collection song: 'Dropping, dropping, dropping,

dropping, hear the pennies fall. Every one for Jesus, Jesus wants them all.' Or was that 'us all'?

Other early screen dogs that come to mind are Ben, Mack Sennett's comedy dog, Pete of *Our Gang*, Asta of *The Thin Man* series, Daisy, so popular in *Blondie* films that 'he' starred in his own movies. Dick Powell was even reincarnated as a handsome German shepherd in *You Never Can Tell*.

There have been scores of dog movies since. A recent trend is for big, shaggy, slobbering dogs creating comedy havoc in fussy households (e.g. *Beethoven*, *Beethoven's 2nd*, *Turner and Hooch*). But no dog films, whether adventure or comedy, can match the international commercial success of the cartoon and live-action permutations of Disney's comedy, *101 Dalmatians*.

Considering the humorous potential of dogs, it's interesting how often the word *dog* or *dogs* in a movie title signifies not comedy – or even the presence of canines – but either appalling luck or extreme violence.

Dog Day and *Dog Day Afternoon* are two films that come to mind in which doomed human characters, respectively an American gangster (Lee Marvin) and an American loser (Al Pacino), have a hellish time of it.

Then there is the adventurous Australian movie *Dogs in Space*, memorable not only for its imaginative examination of the disintegration of the punk subculture (the title refers to the name of a truly terrible punk band), but for starring Michael Hutchence, the lead singer of INXS, later to strangle himself mysteriously in a Sydney hotel room.

Trash-movie buffs might remember the 1964 American-Italian-German co-production *Dog Eat Dog*, starring Jayne Mansfield, a C-grade, unintentionally funny potboiler of lust, depravity and greed in which various characters try to double-cross each other out of a stolen fortune and Jayne constantly complains about her need for clean panties. No one wanted to own up to being *Dog Eat Dog*'s director – and Jayne Mansfield was decapitated in a motor accident shortly after.

But for violence, canine or otherwise, on screen or off, not many films can match Peckinpah's *Straw Dogs* or, on a rising scale of mayhem, Tarantino's *Reservoir Dogs* and the Belgian *cinéma-vérité*, documentary-style satire, *Man Bites Dog*.

Dogs, incidentally, feature in none of these bloodbaths. (Or do I remember the serial killer in *Man Bites Dog* polishing off the family pooch as well as the family?)

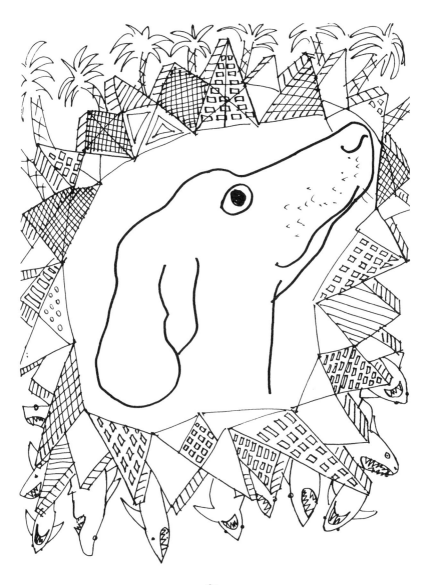

81

The biggest, hairiest 'dog' of a film I've seen in the past few years is *The Island of Dr. Moreau*, the third film version of the famous novel by H.G. Wells, the strangely prescient 'scientific romance' that shocked and scandalised Wells's literary, religious and scientific critics a hundred years ago.

This is a film which tested many people's careers, egos and, indeed, grasps on reality. Much of its considerable curiosity value comes from the on-screen bizarrerie that wasn't in the script. Even if the part the film's star, the gargantuan Marlon Brando, seems to be playing is the balance of nature (or, as Hollywood wisecracked at casting time, the island itself), he can be held only partly responsible for the movie's grotesqueries.

Not only do the beast-people seem to have taken over the movie as well as Dr. Moreau's island, this is a film where the director, Richard Stanley, literally went to the dogs. Stanley, who was sacked by the film's backers only four days into the shoot, then ran off to live in the far North Queensland rainforest with his pet dingo pups – only to return to the set disguised in a Dog-Man costume. He then secretly appeared in the film made by his replacement, the veteran director John Frankenheimer. On this shoot, compared to his colleagues, Brando was a pussycat.

Like Wells's novel and the two earlier Moreau films (with Charles Laughton in 1932 and Burt Lancaster in 1977), the movie tells of a marooned stranger, Douglas (David Thewlis), who stumbles across an obsessed scientist's out-of-control experiments that fuse man with animal.

In the earlier versions, Dr. Moreau's experiments were surgical, conducted in a laboratory which the resulting pathetic monsters called the House of Pain. This Moreau (Brando) is a Nobel Prize-winning geneticist, and the experiments he and his drugged-out assistant, Montgomery (Val Kilmer, very much in character), perform on their zoo of unfortunate animals are to do with gene-splicing, aimed at creating the perfect human being, 'free of all evil impulses'.

If Hyena-Swine, Sow Lady, Boar Man and the other snouted, fanged and horned mutants are anything to go by, the Nobel Committee's standards are slipping. But Moreau holds high hopes for his most successful 'children', the doggish Azazello (Temuera Morrison), the possumish M'Ling (Marco Hofschneider) and the beautiful, almost perfectly human, though tabby-descended Aissa (Fairuza Balk). They alone seem happy standing upright, immune to the general mood of rutting, grunting insolence.

Sole power on the island lies with Moreau. Having embedded an electronic 'pain' chip in every creature's chest, he's able to administer mass shocks by remote control. It takes Hyena-Swine to nut out the pain-chip idea. He's not the best gene-splicing choice, you would think, if the aim is to create a Brad

Pitt with brains, but Hyena-Swine is certainly shrewd enough to tear his chip from his chest. Confronting his god, Moreau, Hyena-Swine asks the anguished question, 'Father, what am I?'

In answer, Moreau tries, unsuccessfully, to shock him. So Hyena-Swine attacks him and kills him.

Considering that his voluminous kaftans have been filling the screen for two-thirds of the film, Moreau's murder is anticlimactic, despite all the snorting and squealing. Predictably, the beast-people revolt, and even those with good table manners start to revert.

They're not the only ones. *The Island of Dr. Moreau* is so over-the-top that even if you wish to ponder, with H.G. Wells, the collision course between the rapid advancement of science and the true evolution of nature, you soon find yourself regressing along with everyone on screen.

(Incidentally, short-time director Stanley is credited only as one of the film's writers. His sneaky Dog-Man appearance goes unmentioned.)

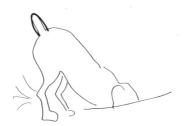

I look up *dog days* in my dictionaries. Collins says *dog days* refers to, firstly, the hot period of the northern summer reckoned in ancient times from the heliacal rising of Sirius (the dog star), and, secondly, to any period marked by inactivity.

The New Shorter Oxford adds that dog days are traditionally regarded as the unhealthiest time of the year, and a period in which malignant influences prevail.

While I'm at it, I count the number of times the New Shorter uses *dog* pejoratively. As a word or prefix to signify contempt, betrayal, disgust, spite, sullenness, ugliness, stupidity, stubbornness or all-round uselessness, *dog* is mentioned ninety-nine times.

Dog is used in a non-pejorative or neutral sense (e.g. dog-weary, dog-tent, dog-collar, dogman) only fifty-two times.

The numbers have it. So what happened to the dog's historical reputation for loyalty and friendship? Historical lexicographers and the modern English language don't seem to believe in it.

The nastiest thing that can be said of a woman is that she's a dog, meaning incredibly unattractive. Of a man, that he's a cat: a sarcastic queen.

This is in line with dogs, whatever their gender, generally being seen as masculine, cats as feminine.

There used to be these cruel competitions, Dog Nights, where young men asked the ugliest girls they knew for a date. When the young women, flattered by this rare male attention, arrived at the party they wondered why all the other females were so homely. Then the penny dropped.

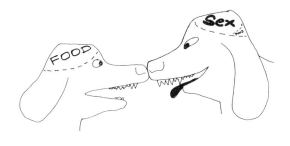

She likes male dogs,
but only if there's
no funny business.
The only trouble she
has is from other
spayed females —
and German shepherds

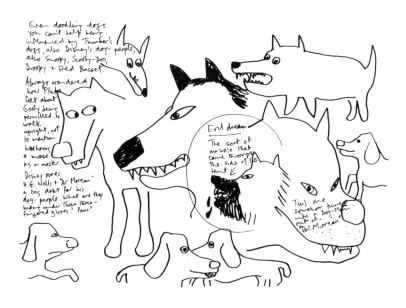

Even doodling dogs
you can't help being
influenced by Thurber's
dogs, also Disney's dog-people,
also Snoopy, Scooby-Doo,
Droopy & Fred Basset.

Always wondered
how Pluto
felt about
Goofy being
permitted to
walk
upright, not
to mention
him having
a mouse
as a master.

Disney owes
H.G. Wells & Dr Moreau
a big debt for his
dog-people. What are they
hiding under those three-
fingered gloves? Paws?

Evil dream:
The sort of
muzzle that
came through
the side of the
tent ↙

This one
somehow turns
into a Dog-Man,
Moreau!

In a male prison (where the cats are the effeminate queens), dogs are held in much lower esteem. A dog, of course, is an informer.

On second thoughts, there is an insult just as bad as calling a man a cat. Calling him a bitch.

On the subject of cats, the poet T.S. Eliot, author of *Old Possum's Book of Practical Cats*, transformed into *Cats*, the stage-musical goldmine for Eliot's publisher Faber & Faber, was actually a dog person. His widow said he preferred them. He once wrote an elegy to a Yorkshire terrier, but nothing theatrical ensued.

As for dogs representing evil, I recall the most frighteningly realistic dream of my life. This was a nightmare about a dog. At the time, in my befuddled, sleepy state, I truly felt I was confronting something supernatural.

The dream was probably caused by a combination of factors. It wasn't too long after we'd acquired Ella and dogs were on my mind. At the time I was finishing writing my novel, *Our Sunshine*, an imaginary life of Ned Kelly, and I'd been concentrating deeply on the last scenes where the police set fire to the Glenrowan pub and ambush its inhabitants, including Ned's brother Dan Kelly and his dog. Dan and Steve Hart are wounded and calling for Ned.

I'd just written:

> *Steve and Dan are staring out. Dan seems to have the*
> *shivers. What now? They've stopped shooting at the police.*
> *All Dan is doing is calling for him, there but not there, in*
> *and out of the fog. Abruptly Dan takes off his helmet and*
> *whistles his dog out, c'mon boy, coaxes it, trembling, from*
> *under the bar, crouches down, who's my old boy, pushes his*
> *face against the muzzle, the dry nose, dry jowls, inhales dry*
> *dog breath, my old boy then.*
>
> *Wants the dog to breathe more on him, fill his lungs,*
> *smother him in breath and slobber. Hugs the dog so hard*
> *it yelps and pulls away.*

At this time I was sleeping out in a tent in the bush behind our house on the Central Coast. The tent was a Christmas acquisition. The children loved camping out, but only if I slept in the tent with them. (There are many scary nocturnal sounds up here.)

And on the first night I dreamed that the muzzle of a ferociously growling dog (or wolf, or fox) was poking through the side of the tent, inches from my face, trying to maul me. I swear I saw it. The frightening thing was that this was happening exactly where I was at that moment, lying on my side facing the tent wall. And I became aware that I was fighting off this snarling dog by bashing at its muzzle with our heavy torch.

I don't know when sleep segued into wakefulness but in the dream I knew this dog was evil, maybe Evil itself. And I woke to find myself sitting up with the torch in my hand, striking the tent wall, shouting fiercely at the dog, in exactly the same position and action as my dream self. Meanwhile, my sleepy son regarded me wonderingly.

Trying to explain this image to myself, I concluded that possums must have been growling and squabbling on a nearby tree stump, which they often do, and that my unconscious had absorbed their growls into the heightened intensity and reality of my dream.

Whatever its causes, the nightmare, or vision, was so strong that I put it in the novel. I gave it to Ned. Dead-tired and weighed down in his body armour, peppered with police bullets in the Glenrowan siege, he hears Dan's panicky dog barking for his dead master.

> *Now he's dreaming, standing. Dreaming of being shot himself, of shattering into a thousand pieces. While he's propped, feet apart for balance, to support the great weight on him, his soul's iron burden, new bullets pop and zing around him, at him, hit him. Somewhere a dog is barking. A dog's head is poking through the side of the hut, as if the wall were air, snout and black lips curling inches from his face. (Joe's snoring, oblivious in the next bunk. Where is this?*

Bullock Creek?) Hello, boy. Why's the dog's pointed muzzle
wrinkled in this snarl of the greatest evil? Long teeth edging
closer. Fear cold as a knife blade flat against his neck.

Listen to me, his mother says, they've got it all wrong.
It's not you that's the very devil, truly, this is it. Shoot the dog.

Muzzle to muzzle, he shoots, and the blast turns it to air.

Talking to her in his head like this, concentrating so deeply
he gets a tingling in his scalp and forehead that fills his skull.
This is hard work, he says to her, sounds like a gulf roaring
in my prickly head. One more thing, am I playing at being
dead, or am I?

A few years after my tent dream, while browsing through
a collection of dog photographs, *Bones,* by the American
photographer Keith Carter, I came across a legend from East
Texas, thought to be African in origin and transplanted to
the Southern culture with the arrival of slaves.

The legend, embodied in countless folktales, tells of a dead
soul returning in the form of a dog to protect and comfort its
loved ones in times of trouble.

Carter's powerful, mysterious, almost primal photographs
recalled a small independent film, *Hannah and the Dog Ghost,*
made by the Texan film-maker Ken Harrison in 1981 as part

of his Texas trilogy. In the film the narrator says: 'When she looked into the eyes of that creature, she knowed what it was. Sure enough, the spirit of her man was beside her now in the shape of a dog. And if there's anything that can give meanness a run for its money, it's a Dog Ghost protecting someone it loves.'

The Swedish poet Artur Lundkvist in his book *Journeys in Dream and Imagination* has described a remarkably similar image (which, coincidentally, also occurred in 1981) after he suffered a heart attack and fell into a coma.

After two months, beginning to slowly emerge into a state of semi-consciousness, he existed in a heightened dream state during which his imagination soared while his body remained immobile and near death.

'It is the dog returning, the same dog or a different one, a shadow dog I cannot clearly perceive. It has no definite form or color, it approaches me somewhat threateningly, with a purpose, but then it becomes uncertain, hesitates, lies down or turns around, starts walking away, but remains silent.'

Hounds, according to the *Dictionary of Sacred Myth*, by Tom Chetwynd, are sometimes three-headed, associated with Hecate, the dark side of the moon, and the underworld, and so with the feminine unconscious and the soul.

They are sometimes related to the planets (was this how Walt Disney came up with Pluto?) and the erratic side of destiny.

In his companion volume, *Dictionary for Dreamers*, Chetwynd says to dream of dogs may relate to the dreamer's attitude to 'dogged' or doglike people: the faithful and devoted companion, or somebody the dreamer can't shake off and who might make trouble (depending on the rest of the dream but also on the dreamer's waking attitude to dogs).

To dream of a dog guarding something is a little more scary and complicated. Chetwynd says the fact that dogs devour corpses may account for their being the guardians of the underworld (Cerberus). These are the hounds of hell, creatures that must be pacified and put to sleep before the dreamer can pass through the underworld.

One winter's evening, jogging along Killcare's wide ocean beach at dusk, the only person on this whole shoreline, I suddenly sensed eyes on me and saw a big black dog staring at me.

It was crouching high up the beach, higher than the winter high-water line, its head up, facing the ocean. The dog's fixed stare and ready-to-spring crouch gave me a start. But with that sinking feeling, so familiar to joggers, of mixed fear, anger and pigheadedness, I kept jogging in its general direction fully expecting it to jump up and chase me.

As I came to within thirty metres of the dog, my heart pumping, I noticed three things about it: it was a big Doberman, its lips were curled in a snarl, and it was dead.

It was an eery sight, lying there in its erect posture – like a lion, like a sphinx – looking out to sea. It was frightening but it was also somehow noble. I kept jogging to the end of the beach, turned, and headed back along the shore. By the time I passed the spot where I'd seen the dead Doberman, the light was too dim, and the beach was strewn with too much dark driftwood, to pick it out from the shoreline. I had no intention of going closer to check it out, and after my exercise I went home.

The next evening my wife and I were walking along the beach and I pointed out where I'd seen the dog. There was no sign of it. But after we'd walked another two or three hundred metres, we looked up the beach, where the dunes met the scrub, and there was the Doberman again, in the same erect crouch, with the same grimace, staring out to sea.

We discussed whether it might have fallen off a yacht and drowned. Or, having swum ashore, then collapsed and died. But why wasn't the body slumped and, well, lifeless? Why was it crouching, head up, in this lifelike way? And why was it positioned higher than the high-tide line? How had it moved overnight? The tide wouldn't have shifted the body in this same watchful pose; it would have rolled it over.

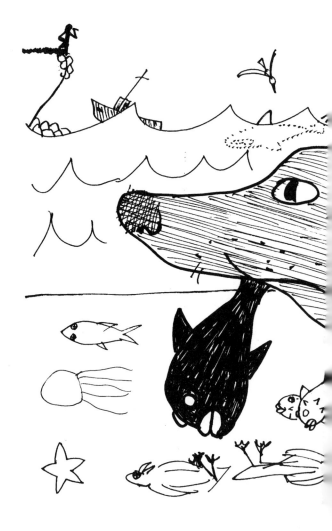

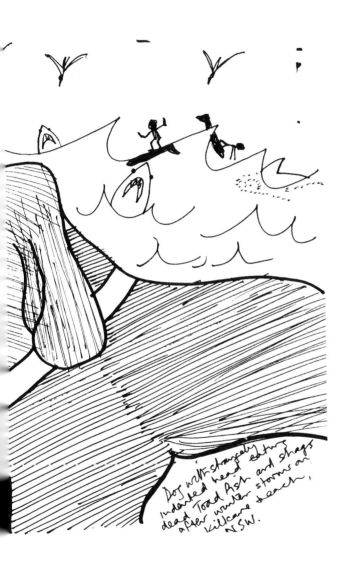

Dog with strange behaviour indarted head eating dead Toad fish and shags after winter storms on Killcare beach, NSW.

Who was it watching for?

Neither of us felt like going closer. Not even a few steps.

Early next morning I was down at the beach again and, in bright daylight, intended to take a closer look at the black dog. There was no sign of it anywhere along the beach. I reasoned that the night's tide must have taken it out to sea again but I wasn't really convinced.

Ella loves to hang around the ragged men who live in the park, even though they hate her. She knows they often have food stashed in the bushes and in the forks of trees and hidden in the windbreaks they make from newspapers and plastic bags and the park benches they've dragged into the shrubbery.

Until recently there was a delicatessen called the Game Kitchen in Oxford Street, Paddington specialising in poultry and game. You could get every table bird there from chicken, duck and goose to pheasant, partridge, squab and even emu.

My eldest daughter worked there (having, as a vegetarian, to daily subdue her nausea during the gutting and dressing) to put herself through university. A group of bearded park-dwelling men used to hang around the Game Kitchen of an afternoon. Before she closed up shop each day, she'd give them any leftover birds. The men would trail back to their hideyholes in the park with their bags of exotic fare.

And on her daily gallop through the park Ella would immediately detect this delicious shift in circumstances and track down the men's bounty. No matter how cleverly they were hidden, how high the tree-fork cache, she'd cart off and dispatch, one by one, each gift parcel of poultry.

This is the only time I've seen her sated with food. So full was she that she'd bury – for later – many of these game birds in the soft garden beds of the mansions bordering the park in Martin Road.

I've sometimes wondered what the owners (or gardeners) of these residences thought when their spades turned up a bag of pheasant or an emu drumstick.

And I've wondered whether my daughter, instead of giving the men the exquisite pleasure and frustration of momentarily possessing a partridge or dressed goose, would have been kinder to eliminate the middle-man (and forestall the violent oaths, the furiously-thrown stones, the unrewarding chase) and bring the leftover birds straight home to Ella.

———————————

Ella is especially attracted to the quiet, bearded park-dweller in the home-made hat. His clothes are made of patches of black leather, rubber and plastic garbage bags sewn together. His hat is a square of black rubber, perhaps an inner tube, with each corner tied in a knot in the manner favoured by English beachgoers and their hankies. Of course Ella is fascinated by his rustling, crackling, rubbery movements.

Each morning, before the garbage trucks come to empty the bins, he gathers and fries a breakfast of leftover picnic scraps on one of the park barbecues. (His frying smells drive Ella crazy.) Then for much of the day he laboriously pedals a heavy black bicycle which is also swathed in leather, rubber and plastic and from whose sides protrudes, among such things as billy cans and briefcases, a garden spade.

The reason for the spade is that he is compelled to chip away any grass which has encroached on the footpath of the park's southern boundary, directly opposite Randwick racecourse, and which spoils its crisp line.

Returning the Randwick footpath to a satisfactory state of straightness can take a whole morning – even longer if a brown dog is constantly sniffing your garments and barking at your rustling trouser cuffs.

The spade was also useful in digging out a sleeping hollow up against the park fence in the patch of bushy waste ground at the Randwick end of Martin Road. For a long while the quiet man in the rubber hat set up a night-time domicile here, he and his bike tucked in for the night directly across the road from some of the grandest residences in Sydney.

The nearest mansion to the sleeping hollow, only fifty metres away from where he hunkered down in the dirt like a wombat, is also the biggest in Martin Road. With its turrets, and wings stretching off to the north and south, it looks like a medieval castle.

Recently some of the rich mansion owners hired a security man to watch over their houses, more specifically to round up those park-dwellers whose lives were beginning to overflow the boundaries of the park.

The security man was known to the park-dwellers as Kiwi Bob. Kiwi Bob soon made his muscular presence felt. He didn't approve of the man in the rubber hat, or his bedroom, and sent him packing.

For many years Patrick White, winner of the Nobel Prize for Literature, lived across the road from the park at 20 Martin Road with his partner Manoly Lascaris and a succession of pug dogs.

White's novella *The Night the Prowler* is a shrewdly evocative story of upper-middle-class Sydney, and specifically an acerbic view of the residents of Martin Road and their deep fear of

This is laughable! Top marks!

Breed	Grooming req.	Temperament	Trainability	Exercise req.	Suitable for
Cattle Dog	Low	Active Excitable	4	High	Adult
Collie	High	Reserved	3	High	Adult Family
Curly Coated Retriever	Medium	Sound	3	Medium	Adult Elderly Family
Dalmatian	Low	Active Excitable Sound	4	High	Adult Family
German Shorthaired Pointer	Low ✓	Active ✓✓✓ Excitable ✓✓	5 !	High ✓✓✓	Adult Family
Golden Retriever	Medium	Sound	5	Medium	Adult Elderly Family
Keeshond	High	Sound	3	Medium	Adult Elderly Family
Kelpie	Low	Active Excitable	5	High	Adult Family
Labrador	Low	Sound	5	Medium	Adult Elderly Family
Samoyed	Medium	Independent Sound	3	Medium	Adult Family
Schnauzer-Standard	Medium Strip	Bold	3	Medium	Adult Family
Shetland Sheepdog	High	Excitable Reserved	4	Medium	Adult Elderly Family
Siberian Husky	Medium	Independent Sound	5	High	Adult Family

cont'd

20

the park's denizens entering their homes in the middle of the night to rape and pillage.

White saw this fear as so ingrained it had become part of their collective unconscious. His characters' bourgeois natures (an unforgivable crime, in his opinion) were unable to cope with the park's anarchic and criminal possibilities.

Jim Sharman's film version of *The Night the Prowler* captured the essence of the story, using the park's shadowy reaches to fine dramatic effect. The film is also remembered for the imaginative casting of its extras, including the distinguished playwright and poet Dorothy Hewett as a ragged, sinister park inhabitant.

White himself loved the park, especially relishing its seedier aspects. His chronic asthma and weather permitting – and rugged up in his woollen beanie cap, scarf and overcoat – he used to walk his pugs there most days.

I saw him there many times, leading and being led by his ugly little dogs around the ponds, but his glare was so fierce and his steps so angrily frail that I couldn't muster the courage to say good day.

To know Patrick White in his Centennial Park heyday carried great social and theatrical cachet and in the mid-1970s the impresario Harry M. Miller, wishing to make a film of *Voss*, bought a mansion nearby. He then brought from London to Centennial Park, in 1976, the distinguished American/British director Joseph Losey (*The Servant* and *The Go-Between*) and the playwright-screenwriter David Mercer, both of whom had White's confidence, to discuss filming the novel and to scout possible locations.

More exciting, from my point of view as a young first-novelist, was Losey's and Mercer's wider reading while in Australia, resulting in their becoming interested in filming *The Savage Crows*, and buying a three-year option for $5000. 'David will be writing it, of course,' said Losey, in case I harboured any such ambitions. But that was fine by me. I was cockahoop.

And I never heard from them again. Mercer's cirrhosis killed him in 1980, and by 1984 Losey, too, was dead. By chance, I met Losey's widow, Patricia, at a party in London in 1989, and my wife and I gave her a lift home. I mentioned that, at one stage at least, *The Savage Crows* had been on her husband's list of forthcoming film projects.

'Funny, Joe never mentioned it,' she said.

After White died on 30 September 1990, having directed in his will that no service or funeral take place to mark his death, and that all his manuscripts be burned, his ashes were scattered in one of the ponds, to be benefit of its hungry eels and bloated carp, its squabbling coots and swamp hens. In the view of his friends, his mordant sense of humour would have found this ending appropriate.

Another muddy Centennial Park pond, the one nearest the junction of Lang and Robertson roads, was the notorious murder scene of Sallie-Ann Huckstepp, whose body was found floating face down in the algae and waterlilies in February 1986.

She was strangled *and* drowned, both forms of violence being given as her cause of death, because she knew too much about the inner workings of Sydney's underworld, especially the convoluted milieu of the city's corrupt police and prominent criminals of that time. No one has ever been convicted of her murder.

Huckstepp, a prostitute and heroin-addict from a middle-class Eastern Suburbs family, was the former lover of the drug dealer and police informer Warren Lanfranchi, who had been shot dead by the disgraced Detective-Sergeant Roger Rogerson five years before. Ever since making allegations about Lanfranchi's death in a television interview, she'd told friends she feared for her life.

Coincidentally, Ced Culbert, the former chief police-rounds reporter on the *Daily Telegraph*, whose reputation rested on his friendship with and loyalty to his police contacts, would later die nearby. In retirement, Culbert suffered a heart attack during his daily constitutional through the park to his favourite watering hole.

———————————————

At the farthest remove from those Centennial Park events was the death in the park of Lady Hailsham, wife of the distinguished British Conservative statesman, who was killed in a horse-riding accident in 1978.

She and her husband, in Sydney for Lord Hailsham to deliver the Sir Robert Menzies Oration at Sydney University, had been riding with two members of the New South Wales mounted police, on horses supplied by the police. Lady Hailsham's horse ('one of the quietest we have,' according to the police) bolted suddenly and she was thrown heavily to the road. She broke her neck and died instantly.

Horrified organisers made it clear that the riding expedition had been arranged at Lord and Lady Hailsham's insistence.

Despite his wife's tragic death, Lord Hailsham insisted on continuing with the Menzies Oration. Chairman of the Conservative Party and a former British Lord Chancellor and Leader of the House of Commons, he had renounced his hereditary title in 1963 (becoming plain Quinton Hogg) in an attempt to win the Prime Ministership. He failed, but was created a life peer in 1970.

Lady Hailsham, aged fifty-eight, was said by the *Evening Standard* to have been 'steeped in Tory politics from an early age, but kept in the background during her husband's career'.

As for the park-dwellers, the park rangers generally don't harass them or move them on. They say the derelicts 'keep an eye on things' for them. Like the notorious flasher who used to expose his 'person' at the Randwick end. And the wealthy flasher who used to do his exposing from the front seat of his burgundy Mercedes.

In the twenty-five years my family has been using the park we've twice fallen victim to park crime. Unfortunately the first time was the only occasion we'd ever been carrying anything valuable: a 21st-birthday-present gold watch and a holiday-pay packet which were foolishly hidden in the car's glovebox – a pleasant surprise for the thief.

The second time was at 7.30 one morning. Apart from early-morning joggers and cyclists the park was almost empty. With our early-rising two-year-old, we were feeding the ducks. While thus engaged and our backs were turned someone stole his stroller, teddy and bottle of milk.

Our watchdog Ella, naturally, was too busy pinching the ducks' bread to notice the thief.

Correction: three crimes. My wife reminds me that the man in the burgundy Mercedes flashed her about ten years ago.

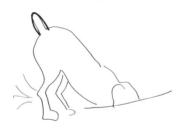

One of the many tensions caused by Ella is everyone's
competing claims to spending vast amounts of quality Ella-
time. Reading these jottings over my shoulder, my wife insists
that she has her own full and close relationship with Ella.
'I love Ella!' she says. Even thinking about Ella makes
people prickly.

When I tell Ella-stories in company she tops them with
one about her driving with Ella and our then baby son to

Bathurst. In this story Ella is let out of the car in the Blue Mountains for urination and exercise, and strews around a bin of baby's disposable nappies and chews up a plastic service-station bucket. When they drive off again my wife checks baby and dog in the rear-vision mirror and Ella is contentedly sucking the baby's dummy.

This is her Ella story and she tells it better than I do. Ella comes across much cuter in her many stories than in mine. No one could deny that canine wellbeing is close to paramount in my wife's mind. As she sets off to work every morning she says, 'Don't forget to walk Ella.' As soon as she's in the door of an evening she's asking, 'Did you walk Ella?' As I mentioned earlier, she is from England.

'Of course,' I say. I've even said it twice when I hadn't, but she could tell.

My daughters scold me. 'You never pat Ella,' they say. 'Give her a cuddle.'

'Of course I do,' I say. 'I cuddle her all day when you aren't here.'

The youngest boy has his own close relationship with Ella. His first words on this earth were 'Bad Dog!'

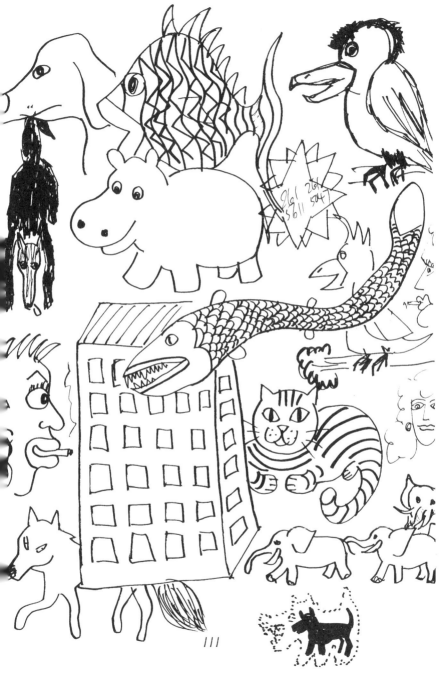

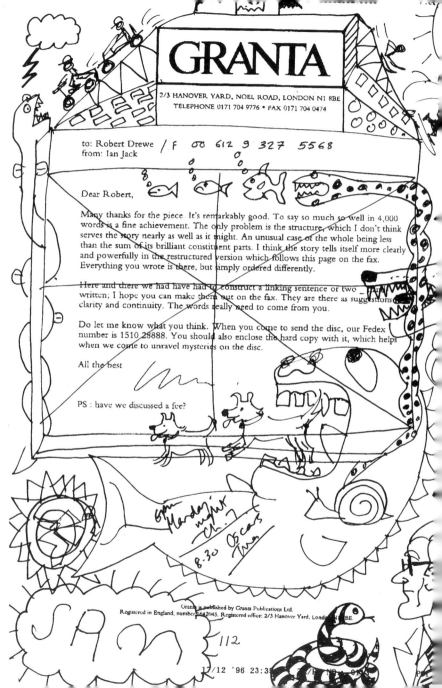

GRANTA

2/3 HANOVER YARD, NOEL ROAD, LONDON N1 8BE
TELEPHONE 0171 704 9776 • FAX 0171 704 0474

to: Robert Drewe / F 00 612 9 327 5568
from: Ian Jack

Dear Robert,

Many thanks for the piece. It's remarkably good. To say so much so well in 4,000 words is a fine achievement. The only problem is the structure, which I don't think serves the story nearly as well as it might. An unusual case of the whole being less than the sum of its brilliant constituent parts. I think the story tells itself more clearly and powerfully in the restructured version which follows this page on the fax. Everything you wrote is there, but simply ordered differently.

Here and there we had have had to construct a linking sentence or two _written; I hope you can make them out on the fax. They are there as suggestions of clarity and continuity. The words really need to come from you.

Do let me know what you think. When you come to send the disc, our Fedex number is 1510 28888. You should also enclose the hard copy with it, which helps when we come to unravel mysteries on the disc.

All the best

PS : have we discussed a fee?

Granta is published by Granta Publications Ltd.
Registered in England, number 1662145. Registered office: 2/3 Hanover Yard, London N1 8BE.

112

17/12 '96 23:3

In summer Ella is allergic to some grasses and bushes in the park and comes out in a rash. She gets itchy lumps as big as ticks in her ears, between her toes, and around her eyes and stomach. She rubs her eyelids on the ground until they bleed and slurps at her genitals so vigorously you feel you should look away or leave the room.

Giving her a cortisone injection, the vet informs me that German shorthaired pointers' skin is sensitive to Australian conditions. I agree, pointing out how the slightest drop in temperature makes her shiver and look miserable, while on hot days she goes limp, sighing and rolling her eyes and casting accusing glances at me, as if I'm responsible for the weather.

'Oh, yes,' says the vet. 'They're great drama queens.'

She's also beginning to get arthritis and once she grew a strange horn on her head like a baby unicorn's. 'Interesting,' said the vet, 'but nothing to worry about.' Indeed, in a month it began to subside and totally vanished.

She has an odd reaction to rain. If she's out on a walk off the lead, or has escaped from the yard, she'll gallop away enthusiastically into the fiercest rainstorm, the wettest shrubbery, the slimiest pond.

But walking on the lead after a brief shower, she'll prissily press herself against the side of the path furthest from the damp grass verge. Even if it's her late-night walk and she's dying to re-mark her territory, she'll resist. She has no intention of letting that nasty wet grass touch her bottom. (I presume the rain has also washed away the other dogs' markings.)

She's also wary of the ocean. The ozone and sand make her skittish but the sea has a sobering effect. Like an old aunt, she'll only paddle up to her knees, and when I dive into the surf she's beside herself with anxiety until I return to the beach. This is the only time she shows any concern for me whatsoever so I find it quite endearing.

In bookshops these days I find myself strangely drawn to dog books.

I feel as self-conscious perusing them as if I'm browsing through hardcore porn. I also feel self-indulgent buying them.

But then if I hadn't read *Leader of the Pack* I'd still be politely holding the door open for everyone, people and dogs alike, and never have taken the necessary steps towards gaining my Alpha Wolf status.

Many of the books are so sentimental and anthropomorphic they make your fillings ache. More man's-best-friend stuff. This is why *Knitting with Dog Hair* stands out. I thought this must be a spoof, but no. Its American female authors, Kendall Crolius and Anne Black Montgomery, while appearing to be a few pups short of a litter, take their subject very seriously. This book is a labour of love.

Ms Crolius, we're told, has been spinning yarn from her pets' hair and knitting her clothes with it for most of her life. As she holds down a job as senior vice president at J. Walter Thompson, this must have caused the occasional wisecrack on Madison Avenue over the years. Ms Montgomery is a writer on 'dogs and home-making' for *Town & Country*.

Of course the most informative chapter is 'The Spinner's Guide to Dog Breeds'. Naturally I couldn't wait to see what sort of a garment I could knit out of a German shorthaired pointer's moultings. Alas, as in many areas, Ella falls short. According to the authors: 'A weekly grooming will yield little worth spinning. Sprinkle the fallen hairs with less difficult fibres and point with pride to the finished product – a camouflage scarf, perhaps.'

What you really need is an Afghan hound, Samoyed, collie, golden retriever, Irish setter, English sheepdog – a dog of ample hairiness. The good news for nationalists is that Australian silky-terrier hair makes a very presentable sweater.

———————————

When the British author and animal-observer Desmond Morris produced two companion volumes, *Dogwatching* and *Catwatching*, he found that the latter outsold the former two to one. *Catwatching* was even discovered selling well at dog shows.

Given that the British are famous dog-owners, and that in Britain there are approximately six million dogs and six million cats, the author Julian Barnes has worried about this dichotomy. He has pondered whether (a) cat-owners are more literate, (b) cat-owners all live in city flats with the latest paperbacks while dog-owners live down muddy lanes miles from the nearest bookshop, (c) there is some connection between curling up with a cat and curling up with a book, (d) dog-exercising is a thorough psychological substitute for reading, (e) cats like the quiet rustle of a turning page while dogs prefer the more vigorous stimulation of television, (f) dogs bully their owners into not reading, and (g) dogs eat books.

Incidentally, 66 per cent of Australian households have a pet, and 68 per cent of these pet-owners have one or more dogs.

Eighty per cent of children who are bitten by dogs are bitten in their own homes. Forty-three per cent are under five.

On the subject of the conjunction of dogs and literature, the cultured and elegant hostess of a national television books programme makes the acquaintance of Ella while spending a weekend at our coastal shack in the bush.

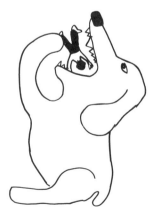

The TV hostess, unused to either children or animals, has been regarding both our boisterous twelve-month-old son and our boisterous dog, not to mention her surroundings, with the alternate detachment, surprise and curiosity of the European urbanite abruptly transported to, say, white-trash rural Arkansas.

So it's with smothered giggles that my wife and I suddenly notice the neat line of pellets which our small naked boy is leaving across the hearth. Just as it is with mortified embarrassment that, following the TV hostess's horrified and fascinated gaze, we see Ella chasing and gobbling up the pellet trail.

———————

The growth area in dog publishing is dog psychology. The titles say it all: *The Hidden Life of Dogs*, *The Dog Who Loved Too Much*, *The Dog's Mind*, *The Intelligence of Dogs*, *Minds of Their Own*, *Thinking in Pictures*.

In her runaway bestseller *The Hidden Life of Dogs*, the author, Elizabeth Marshall Thomas, announces: 'I would like to know what the world looks like to a dog, or sounds like, or smells like. I would like to visit a dog's mind – to have another dog look at me and see not something different but something the same.'

Then she poses the Big Question (the one asked by the ruling class of all impatient minorities): What do dogs want?

In some of these books sentimentalism and science seem to be in direct conflict. Scientist-authors dedicate their books to their Rhodesian ridgebacks or simultaneously acknowledge their literary agents and their Jack Russells.

But thinking about consciousness in animals gets me thinking. These writers are asking whether animals have ideas, and whether they think about objects they can't see or about situations that have occurred in the past. They're asking whether dogs and chickens and gorillas are consciously making plans for the future or simply reacting unthinkingly to objects as they appear and to situations as they arise.

I must say that the idea of visiting Ella's mind is not the slightest bit engaging. Am I impossibly arrogant, indeed a species fascist, in imagining that I know quite well what Ella wants (food, food, food, then shelter and affection), in believing that she hasn't exactly been hiding her secret longings from me?

But then I'm as positive as most dog-owners would be that she has ideas, and that she mulls over situations from the past. (German-shepherd attacks? Drunks lurching at her outside the Windsor Castle pub? The Dog and Master Obedience School?)

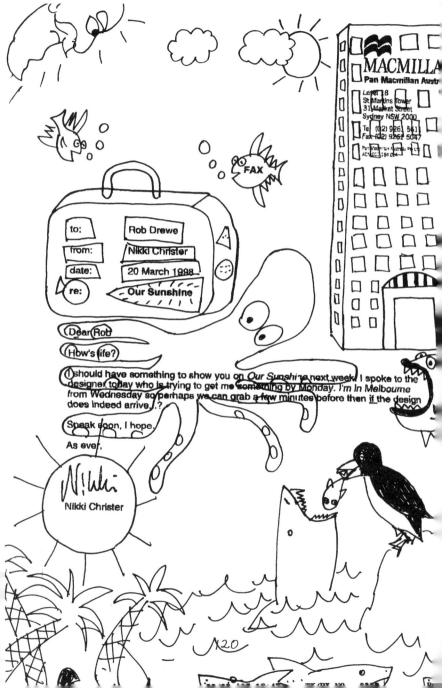

MACMILLAN
Pan Macmillan Aust.

Level 18
St. Martins Tower
31 Market Street
Sydney NSW 2000

Tel (02) 9261 5611
Fax (02) 9261 5047

Pan Macmillan Australia Pty Ltd
ACN 003 184 014

to: Rob Drewe

from: Nikki Christer

date: 20 March 1998

re: Our Sunshine

Dear Rob

How's life?

I should have something to show you on *Our Sunshine* next week. I spoke to the designer today who is trying to get me something by Monday. I'm in Melbourne from Wednesday so perhaps we can grab a few minutes before then if the design does indeed arrive...?

Speak soon, I hope.

As ever,

Nikki Christer

Elizabeth Marshall Thomas says she knows what dogs want. They want each other.

'Human beings are merely a cynomorphic substitute. Dogs who live in each other's company are calm and pragmatic, never showing the desperate need to make known their needs and feelings or to communicate their observations, as some hysterical dogs who know only the company of our species are likely to do. Dogs who live in each other's company know they are understood.'

That sounds perfectly reasonable. But then why did dogs all those years ago choose to leave the wolf pack to live with us?

The sample dogs on which she bases her thesis are two Siberian huskies and a dingo. Is this sample big enough? And who would say that these particular animals, being hundreds of generations closer to their wolf origins, were representative of the world's domestic dogs in the twenty-first century?

The American archaeologist Professor Bob Wayne has found that dogs have been with us far longer than the fifty thousand years that archaeology suggests. His findings? One hundred thousand years. 'We have evolved together.'

———————

I must admit to knowing what at least one dog wanted. This was Charlie, better known as Puppy. Puppy was the dog of my former marriage. What he wanted was to run away and join the circus.

Puppy was a sportsman, a gymnast, an athlete. He was a medium-sized, good-natured, amazingly agile black mongrel. He could run straight up and over a three-metre-high fence. He was conditioned to chase and catch, and did these things as reflexively as any Test cricket fieldsman. He always caught tennis balls on the first bounce. (He anticipated the angle of ricochet.) If you put a stick on top of a playground slippery-dip, he would climb the metal ladder, pick up the stick and slide down, grinning, with the stick in his mouth.

He was never home. Because he was easily able to scale that three-metre back fence, he would do so. Every day. Mostly I'd find him down in the park, leading a merry band of similarly minded scoundrels. But, *pace* Ella, when I whistled, he would stop what he was doing and tear towards me. Even when he was having fun he loved to see me appear.

He was the Shep I never had. He was a ten-year-old's dream dog. Unfortunately I was thirty.

He loved me, he loved the family, but he was a genuine wanderer, as much at the mercy of his genes and glands as the protagonists in *The Hidden Life of Dogs*. You'd glimpse him from the car four kilometres from home, performing tricks for strange children in a block of flats, or walking purposefully along the harbour wall. He and his lightning reflexes were also at the mercy of the five cackling teenagers next door, who'd whistle him over the fence and incite him to ever greater risks by throwing balls into the traffic or into the harbour.

But he was, just barely, at home in his near-city environment. Except the more he went out and the worse company he kept, the harder he was to control (once he'd apologetically eaten and drunk and slept for twenty-four hours) when he was at home. When a tough old spayed bitch taught him to chase cars, he was hooked, and Lesson Number One and our last vestige of discipline disappeared.

And so I found myself in the haunting, never-anticipated position of sending a dog to the country.

This, however, was the genuine country, a farmlet west of Sydney, on whose fifty acres Puppy's skills and energy would be better tested than in a four-metre-wide terrace house. Of course it was kinder. The way his life was going, the way he was burning the candle at both ends, my – our – decision would almost certainly prolong it.

Thus I convinced myself. In those days, at a time when I had other, pressing, human things on my mind, it was a shockingly easy decision to make. Strange then, that the old belief has lately resurfaced. That to be 'sent to the country' really meant to be sentenced to death.

I find it difficult to talk about Puppy. I feel a strong guilt about him. What did I think I was doing?

For those of us who still find the idea of dog psychology a teensy bit precious, Dr Lesley Rogers in *Minds of Their Own* reminds sceptics that only three and a half centuries ago Descartes and others were advocating the view that animals were machines, differing from human-made machines only in their degree of complexity.

According to the Cartesian view, the yelping of a beaten dog was merely the creaking of the animal's clockwork machinery. Today who would disagree that all vertebrate animals, at least, can feel pain?

After reading all this Dog-Shrink Lit, I come to the strange realisation that Ella seems remarkably well-adjusted.

Compared to a blanket-sucking dachshund, a springer spaniel with rage syndrome, an anxiety-attacked Afghan or a golden retriever with obsessive-compulsive disorder she seems, well, almost normal.

All these case-histories, and others (Rocky, the ferocious Rottweiler; Tammy, the collie with a fear of Thursdays; Sybil, the German shepherd terrified of thunder; and of course Elsa, the labrador who loved too much) are examined in *The Dog Who Loved Too Much*, by Dr Nicholas Dodman.

The book's title relates to separation anxiety. Dogs that suffer the condition, says Dr Dodman, bark and whine and wreak havoc in their owners' absence because they're the product of their environment, the canine equivalent of a dysfunctional person. They lack self-esteem and live vicariously through their owners, whom they adore and on whom they're totally dependent.

He tells the famous story of the faithful English gun dog that was inadvertently locked in the parlour during its owners' lengthy absence. The dog didn't eat any of the plentiful food surrounding it and died of starvation, obedient to the end.

'Although this is an inspiring, though pathetic, story of seeming altruism, another explanation is equally moving: separation anxiety, a cardinal feature of which is anorexia – to the bitter end.'

What's to blame for this terrible anxiety and anorexia? Psychological trauma in early puppyhood. Dr Dodman says dogs with separation anxiety often have a dog-pound or pet-store history, or come from a person who didn't spend much time with them. They've been mistreated through isolation and neglect, and (enter, Freud!) may have been separated from their mothers and litter-mates too early.

He says separation anxiety can be predicted with one hundred per cent accuracy in pound dogs, based on the reason the dog was brought to the pound in the first place and compounded by the fact that they were.

But the scenario guaranteed to produce canine separation anxiety, says Dr Dodman, is the impersonal rearing of batches of dogs in the puppy mills of the US Midwest. In these breeding farms, puppies are separated from their mothers at the tender age of four or five weeks and transported many miles to their destination, the pet stores, where they're handled extensively, but only by an assortment of complete strangers. Pet-store dogs are usually sold when they're between three and five months old, after spending months in isolation during a critical period of their social development.

'The product? Little Orphan Annie in a dog suit – an accident looking for a place to happen. If the new owners are kindly people, the dog will cling to them like the proverbial drowning man will clutch at a straw.'

Coincidentally, the *Guardian Weekly* today tells how a 1982 British Government scheme urging Welsh dairy farmers to breed dogs as a way of supplementing income hurt by dwindling milk quotas has resulted, twenty-four years later, in the multi-million-pound industry of illegal puppy farms.

Not given to tabloid-style sob-stories, the *Guardian* reveals the existence of hundreds of puppy farms, mostly converted cowsheds, cramped, dirty, dark and rife with disease. Hereditary diseases are passed on by exhausted bitches which, like battery hens, are mated as often as possible, producing two or three litters a year. Some, says the *Guardian*, are held down by pitchforks to be forcibly mated.

It's a lucrative business. Three Welsh areas alone – Carmarthenshire, Ceredigion and Pembrokeshire – have 260 licensed dog breeders and 500 unlicensed breeders, according to the RSPCA. The Kennel Club estimates that 420 000 farmed puppies are bred and sold each year. The average price of a pedigree puppy is 250 pounds.

Owners may not get what they pay for. Pneumonia, pleurisy, diarrhoea, worms, skeletal deformations and big vets' bills can come included in the price.

The puppies are products, bought and sold for profit, exported and bred to order. Credit card in hand, a British buyer can phone the nearest dial-a-dog dealer, express a preference, say, for a King Charles spaniel, and wait for delivery, just like pizza. Buyers in Japan, Hong Kong and Taiwan, where increasing numbers of puppies are exported, will pay more than 1000 pounds each.

———————————

Dog faeces is lately as much on one's mind in any inner-city residential area as it used to be (and let's face it, still is) on one's shoes.

The new, socially-conscious act of collecting your dog's faeces in a plastic bag is not an unqualified success around our way. I've noticed that dog-owners, having conscientiously collected their pet's deposits, are then leaving the sealed bags in the gutter.

In a recent downpour, the sight of a dozen air-tight bags of dog shit sailing down the hill towards Sydney Harbour was cause for contemplation. Is it intended that Bruno's and Fifi's crap be preserved for posterity?

———————————

Another reminder to the Alpha Wolf from *Leader of the Pack*: 'The leader of the pack always eats first. That is his right. It indicates to those in and out of the pack just who the leader is.

Let him see you eat, from a position at least six to ten feet away. If your dog does not know how to stay in a spot on command or becomes too excited or pushy and can't stay away from your table, put on his leash and tether him to a doorknob in sight of your dinner table. Then ignore him while you enjoy your meal, even if he begins to bark or whine.

If the barking gets out of hand, however, get a spray bottle, fill it with water, set it on a tight stream, and spray Bobo right in the face, from where you are sitting. When you spray the dog, simultaneously say No! and then Quiet!

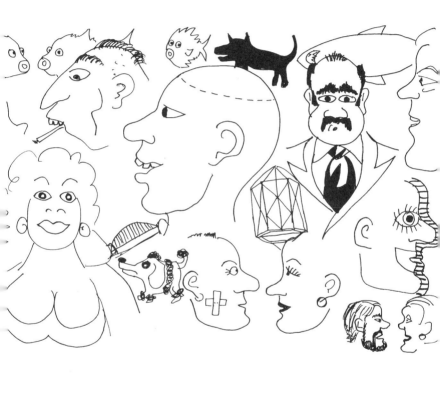

Continue eating, and repeat the spraying if necessary, unless your dog enjoys the squirt of water. This works for some dogs and not others. You may also try a loud, sudden sound. Do not lose your temper or give in to the dog. Adopt an attitude of stoic indifference.'

———————

My stars on the other hand, according to 'Your Capricorn Pet' in the *Sunday Telegraph*, suggest that I should never have become involved with a German shorthaired pointer in the first place.

'Capricorns are hardy, independent and protective, and their ideal pet should reflect those qualities. The labrador is a dog of good character, an excellent family pet that thrives in the spacious environment usually enjoyed by their Capricorn owner.

The British Blue cat, which has dignity and a gentle disposition, is a favourite, and goats, depicted in the symbol of Capricorn, are naturally compatible. Pets to watch rather than play with, such as rabbits, which create their own homes, and tortoises, which carry homes on their back, tickle a Capricorn's fancy.'

So, I can be truly content only if I allow a goat, a tortoise, a rabbit, a blue cat and a labrador into my life.

———————

Surprisingly, to my way of thinking, a friend, the playwright and novelist Louis Nowra, finds himself wonderfully compatible with chihuahuas. Interviewed by Candida Baker for her *Yacker* series of interviews with Australian writers, Louis discussed the births of his dogs.

'The vet was so drunk that my wife (the composer Sarah de Jong) and I had to perform the caesarian with the vet instructing us, and when the puppies were born we had to give them the kiss of life.

When Sarah and I were divorced we determined the custody of the dogs by going to opposite ends of the house and calling them by name. Candy and Brutus went to me, and Iggy and Lulu went to Sarah. There are occasional family reunions.'

When Pope John Paul II came to Sydney in 1995 thousands of the Catholic faithful, including the then Australian Prime Minister, Paul Keating, flocked to Randwick racecourse to see him and to receive God's love through him.

Centennial Park of course is just across the road from the racecourse. Attracted by the smell of the food stalls set up just inside the gates, Ella interrupted our walk, shot across the road through the traffic and police cordons and vanished into the crowd. When I last spotted her she was trotting along, holding what looked like a big piece of Lebanese bread.

The Pope's security was an issue at the time. Dishevelled, and wearing shorts and running shoes, I was turned back by police when I tried to get her. There was nothing to do but go home.

She arrived home a couple of hours later looking soulful but bloated, drank two bowls of water, repaired to the sofa and passed out. We could only hope she'd been included in the Pontiff's blessing.

Incidentally, I saw on TV that Paul Keating had given his children a German shorthaired pointer for Christmas. Before long there were leaks to the Press from his disgruntled domestic staff complaining that the dog demanded too much attention. It was either too cold or too hot and required a specially heated and cooled kennel. It was costing taxpayers money. It was untrainable and creating havoc at The Lodge.

Newsclips showed it eating as if its life depended on it.

Paul Keating lost the next election in a landslide to the Liberal-National Party coalition. I blame the dog.

The Ella.

In the eight years since the first edition of this dossier on Ella was published her notoriety has spread. Hearing me calling her name in public, dog-walking strangers sometimes stop in their tracks and inquire, 'That's not *the* Ella?'

They stare at her with expectant frowns, waiting for her to eat a dead pelican or terrorise someone in a sari. They expect her to look more interesting than a mere brown dog wandering through the park or nosing along a beach sniffing bluebottles.

I'm not sure whether to be embarrassed or pleased. I was, however, intrigued to discover that *the* Ella was indeed the subject of an entire chapter ('A Dog Down Under') in a recent British book, *One Dog and His Man*, by the author and dog-lover Trevor Grove.

Mr Grove courteously sent me a copy of his book, which acknowledges *Walking Ella* as an influence. A Londoner, his dog-walking beat is Hampstead Heath, whose wildlife (apart from some idiosyncratic mating humans) is limited to squirrels and rabbits. He says that Ella, with her wider and more exotic choice of park foodstuffs, is 'a far more heroic guzzler' than his dog. Moreover, Beezle, a male Dalmatian with a nose for sexual foreplay rather than non-stop food, seems like a pleasant, normal dog.

As an intemperate, bohemian sort of dog, Ella, of course, has always lived life on the edge. Until recently. She is now fifteen years old. This fact astonishes me every day, as it does everyone who knows her. No one – least of all her family – ever expected her to reach double figures.

Apart from her dangerous wandering habits and toxic meal choices she has survived at least two life-threatening occurrences. The first was being rounded up and savaged by two German shepherds, working in coldly efficient unison, in Centennial Park. (She needed sixty stitches and was hospitalised for a week.) The second was being knocked unconscious by a hit-and-run taxi in Randwick.

She was lucky to be helped by a kind young Chinese student who had witnessed the incident. Aided by a block of Cadbury's fruit and nut chocolate from his backpack, he brought her around. He didn't know that chocolate is supposedly poison to dogs. Though not in Ella's case, where it acted like a whiff of smelling salts. She scoffed the lot and was her normal self in no time.

But there is no getting away from the fact that Ella is now old. As is often the way – with humans as well as dogs – she became old quite abruptly. Until she was thirteen she was as footloose and fancy-free as ever. Two things seemed to suddenly age her: the onset of arthritis and New Year's Eve 2003.

Because of her fearful reaction to New Year fireworks we'd always kept her shut indoors as midnight approached. This time the fireworks began much earlier. In a lull between explosions, during the arrival of guests, she slunk outside and sped off into the night.

Our New Year's Eve party broke up into a frustrating neighbourhood search for Ella. Finally, at 4 a.m., came an irate phone call from the sleepless owners of our old house. Two years after we'd moved, Ella had turned up there, howling and barking. She couldn't be encouraged inside, they said, nor would she be shooed away or quietened. Indeed, I could hear her frantic barking over the phone.

When I arrived, she darted towards me, then dashed away, barking dementedly. She kept this up at a high pitch. Inside, the new householders were muttering and cursing and stamping about. I called and cajoled. It had been a long night and now, in the dark pre-dawn, a New Year's hangover looming, I was chasing this canine lunatic around the yard of a house where we no longer lived.

Perhaps thirty minutes passed. Ella was still behaving crazily. It was impossible to catch her. I could sense a neighbourhood rebellion brewing around us. A faint light appeared in the sky and the first kookaburras of the new year began expressing themselves.

Tired and exasperated, I slumped down in my old yard. And this surprised her. Perhaps she thought I had died of fatigue and mortification. She stopped barking and sprinting in mad circles around the house and approached this familiar human collapsed on the grass. She gave me a curious sniff, as if to say, 'What on earth are *you* doing here?' I put her on the leash and we drove home into the new year.

After that fright she ceased to wander. She has stuck close to home ever since.

Ella has turned into an old lady, somewhere between a sort of horizontal brown grandma and an ageing showgirl. She snorts and wheezes around the house, and when she needs a door opened for her she no longer waits patiently to enter or depart, but howls an abject dog-word which sounds like 'Owen!'

She feels the cold, and favours a green coat with Velcro straps to keep her snug. While it is being put on her she stands quite still and makes a satisfied clicking sound, as if she's adjusting her dentures. Her nails are growing quicker and longer now, and she's losing her eyesight and hearing. In her green jacket and long nails she totters and taps around the house, for all the world like an old actress in stilettos.

She first started going grey at the muzzle. The grey began at the nose and lips then spread outwards and upwards to the eyebrows. Now it's spread even to her paws and chest. And whitened. Her liver colour has faded in patches on her haunches, like a rug that gets too much sun.

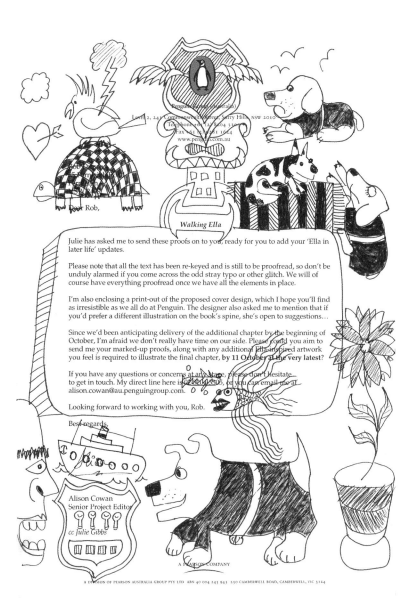

Penguin Group (Australia)
Level 2, 247 Commonwealth Street, Surry Hills, NSW 2010
Telephone +61 (2) 8204 3100
Fax +61 (2) 8204 1624
www.penguin.com.au

Walking Ella

Dear Rob,

Julie has asked me to send these proofs on to you, ready for you to add your 'Ella in later life' updates.

Please note that all the text has been re-keyed and is still to be proofread, so don't be unduly alarmed if you come across the odd stray typo or other glitch. We will of course have everything proofread once we have all the elements in place.

I'm also enclosing a print-out of the proposed cover design, which I hope you'll find as irresistible as we all do at Penguin. The designer also asked me to mention that if you'd prefer a different illustration on the book's spine, she's open to suggestions…

Since we'd been anticipating delivery of the additional chapter by the beginning of October, I'm afraid we don't really have time on our side. Please could you aim to send me your marked-up proofs, along with any additional Ella-inspired artwork you feel is required to illustrate the final chapter, **by 11 October at the very latest**?

If you have any questions or concerns at any stage, please don't hesitate to get in touch. My direct line here is 02 8204 3305, or you can email me at alison.cowan@au.penguingroup.com.

Looking forward to working with you, Rob.

Best regards,

Alison Cowan
Senior Project Editor

cc Julie Gibbs

A PEARSON COMPANY

A DIVISION OF PEARSON AUSTRALIA GROUP PTY LTD ABN 40 004 245 943 250 CAMBERWELL ROAD, CAMBERWELL, VIC 3124

She often jumps up, barking furiously at a family member entering the room, then sleeps soundly through the thumping and clanking arrival of a team of tradesmen-strangers with buckets and ladders. She moans 'Owen!' to come in, and 'Owen!' to go out. She sees ghost dogs in the hallway.

The vet says to limit her walks to ten minutes a time. As well as arthritis in her hips she has bursitis in a front leg joint. Ella has *tennis elbow*.

Lately she has taken to sleeping under my desk. She is lying by my feet – a sentimental touch – as I write this. It occurs to me that a normal dog would do this, too. Suddenly I remember the morning fourteen years ago when a bemused inner-city stranger phoned to say tersely, 'Your dog is upstairs asleep on my bed.'

These days we live on the far north coast of New South Wales. I'm not sure if Ella misses the city but she has no time for horses or cows and gives them a wide berth. (Although occasionally she might fancy a quick horse-manure snack.) She is scared of the family rabbit, whose macho aggression unnerves her. At night we keep her inside in case she tries to eat a poisonous cane toad.

She is still attracted to bizarre foodstuffs, but now she buries them deeply and thriftily, like a squirrel. Currently her garden-larder includes three mouldy slices of bread, a hambone and a fatally window-concussed parrot. She has not lost her sense of smell in the slightest. Or her constant hunger.

During our daily beach walk she still eschews the sea, except for an ankle-deep paddle on hot days. Notwithstanding that she's supposed to be a water-dog, she has attempted to swim only twice in her life, in the same placid rock pool. But only because the whole family was frolicking there and she thought she was missing out on something.

No matter how thirsty she is, she won't drink fresh running water. Frustratingly, even on the hottest of days she will never drink either from the tap or from any receptacle beneath it. The surface of her water bowl has to be motionless. Despite this phobia she'll drink stagnant algae-encrusted pond water. After several thousand beach visits she still laps up seawater – and then acts surprised at the taste.

Often at Seven Mile Beach she and I stop to watch a local golden retriever body-surfing. The retriever enjoys itself surfing waves into shore, then catching the undertow, riding the 'gutter' out again, just like a human surfer. Its owner stands proudly by. Ella, rather shamefaced, changes the subject by urinating on the nearest sandy protuberance, as if to obliterate the retriever's existence.

Occasionally she loses me at the beach. She's apt to panic these days. When this happens – because her sight is going –

I have to run upwind of her so she can smell me. If she's very confused I take off my shirt and wave it in the breeze. She can detect and differentiate my body odour at about five hundred metres. I'm not sure how proud I should be of this.

———————————

I am proud, however, of one particular Sunday in Centennial Park. This day, as the result of some increased sternness of attitude by the Centennial Park administration, the park is suddenly covered with signs – some brusque, some informative to the nth degree.

Big patches of the park are suddenly dry and brown. Signs say 'Noxious Weed Removal (i.e. poison). This area is being cleared of noxious weed. The removal programme involves six species, including lantana, blackberry and pampas grass.'

Other signs warn walkers about the branches of coral trees falling on their heads ('They are in decline and dangerous'), or warn drivers of the severe fines for driving over 30 kmh.

In the area of the park where dogs are allowed to run free there are new signs saying 'Dogs Must Be Under Control'. This is rather like putting up a sign saying, 'Men Must Be Rich'. To be earnestly desired but not in the realm of possibility.

How to be simultaneously free and under control is the problem.

During this period of increased park-ranger officiousness, a female ranger screeches to a halt in her four-wheel drive and approaches me when I'm in the middle of a park dilemma.

My four-year-old, a long way from a lavatory, is mortified at having had an accident in his pants. I'm kneeling in the pampas grass trying to deal with it. At the same time, Ella has just discovered half a dead possum fifty metres away, a strip of rigid fur and bones, and is beginning to munch it.

'Control your dog!' the ranger shouts.

'In a minute,' I say, looking up. Oh, God. 'Anyway, she's not out of control. She's standing quite still, eating.'

'She's eating a possum!' says the ranger.

'A dead possum,' I point out, over my little boy's embarrassed wails. He's dragging me towards the car to cover his mess and shame, to get him quickly home.

'That possum could be alive!' says the ranger.

'But it isn't.'

'Don't walk off while I'm talking to you!' shouts the ranger, confusing herself with a police inspector.

'It's as stiff as a board. It's as flat as a pancake. It's been run over by a car. It stinks. It hasn't got a head. It's been dead for weeks. You're not suggesting she killed it?'

'Well,' says the ranger, revealing an ignorance of dogs' bizarre fondness for meat, 'she shouldn't be eating it. Women and children don't like to see that sort of thing.'

I can't help wildly glancing around and asking, 'What women and children? Where?'

Why this gender favouritism? Why these sheltered sensibilities? Is she talking about herself?

'Control your dog!' the ranger yells. 'Or I'll take your name and address. You don't have control of your dog!'

And this rapidly escalating episode, somewhere between *Catch-22* and *Monty Python*, suddenly comes to a conclusion.

Tense and harassed, I give one sharp whistle. Ella drops the cadaver like a hot coal, sprints towards me and leaps – like a perfectly trained circus dog, like a dog in a dog-food commercial, like heroic Lassie or Rin Tin Tin – onto the back seat of the car.

And although the car's interior is gaggingly pungent, what with Ella panting her carcass-breath down my neck and my child's accident seeping into the upholstery, it's with a rare light heart, not to mention the quiet pride of the dog-owner, that I drive out through the park gates.

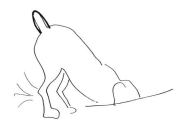

Further Reading

The following books were either mentioned in *Walking Ella* and/or perused as part of my trying to fathom her behaviour. Some did indeed provide a deeper understanding of dogs, some were diverting, entertaining, humorous or irritating, many were 'heart-warming', most (isn't it the way?) say more about their author-owners than they do about dogs. Or cats.

Baer, Nancy, and Duno, Steve, *Leader of the Pack* (HarperCollins, 1996)

Baker, Candida, *The Powerful Owl* (Picador, 1994)

——*Yacker 3: Australian Writers Talk About Their Work* (Picador, 1989)

Carter, Keith, *Bones* (Chronicle Books, 1996)

Chetwynd, Tom, *Dictionary for Dreamers* (HarperCollins, 1993)

——*Dictionary of Sacred Myth* (HarperCollins, 1994)

Crolius, Kendall, and Montgomery, Anne, *Knitting with Dog Hair* (Hutchinson, 1996)

Dodman, Nicholas, *The Dog Who Loved Too Much* (Bantam, 1996)

Drewe, Robert, *The Bay of Contented Men* (Penguin, 2001)

——*Our Sunshine* (Penguin, 2001)

——*The Savage Crows* (Penguin, 2001)

Grove, Trevor, *One Dog and His Man* (Atlantic Books, 2003)

'The Hobyahs' from *The Second Victorian Reader* (Victorian Government Printer, 1930)

Holmes, Charles S., *The Clocks of Columbus: The Literary Career of James Thurber* (Secker & Warburg, 1973)

Kriegel, Volker, *The Truth About Dogs* (Bloomsbury, 1998)

Lawson, Henry, *The Penguin Henry Lawson: Short Stories* (Penguin, 1986)

McCarty, Diane, *German Shorthaired Pointers* (THF Publications, 1996)

Marshall Thomas, Elizabeth, *The Hidden Life of Dogs* (Weidenfeld and Nicolson, 1994)

New Yorker magazine and Mitchell, Carolyn B., *The New Yorker Book of Dog Cartoons* (Knopf, 1992)

Pinker, Steven, *How the Mind Works* (Allen Lane, 1998)

Pitcher, George, *The Dogs Who Came to Stay* (Weidenfeld and Nicolson, 1996)

Rogers, Lesley J., *Minds of Their Own* (Allen & Unwin, 1997)

Sebring Lowry, Janet, and Tenggren, Gustaf, *The Poky Little Puppy* (Golden Books, 1942)

Steinbeck, John, *Travels with Charley: In Search of America* (Penguin, 1980)

Weston, David and Ruth, *Your Ideal Dog* (Hyland House, 1997)

White, Patrick, *The Night the Prowler* (Penguin, 1978)

VIKING

Published by the Penguin Group
Penguin Group (Australia)
250 Camberwell Road, Camberwell, Victoria 3124, Australia
(a division of Pearson Australia Group Pty Ltd)

Penguin Books Ltd, Registered Offices: 80 Strand, London WC2R 0RL, England

First published by Box Press Pty Ltd, 1998
This edition published by Penguin Group (Australia),
a division of Pearson Australia Group Pty Ltd, 2006

10 9 8 7 6 5 4 3 2 1

Cover designed by Jay Ryves © Penguin Group (Australia)
Text designed by Cheryl Collins Design
Illustrations by Robert Drewe
Cover illustration by Robert Drewe
Typeset in 11/15 pt Goudy by Post Pre-press Group, Brisbane, Queensland
Printed and bound in China through Bookbuilders

National Library of Australia
Cataloguing-in-Publication data:

Drewe, Robert, 1943– .
    Walking Ella : ruminations of a reluctant dog-walker.

    Bibliography.
    ISBN 0 670 02962 9.

    1. Drewe, Robert, 1943– . 2. Dogs – Anecdotes. 3. Dog walking – Anecdotes.
    4. Dog owners – Anecdotes. 5. Human–animal relationships. I. Title.

636.7

www.penguin.com.au